Nursing Research
Text and Workbook

Fourth Edition

Patricia Ann Dempsey, R.N., Ph.D.

Professor of Nursing, New Mexico State University,
Las Cruces, New Mexico

Arthur D. Dempsey, Ed.D.

Gadsden, New Mexico, School District

Little, Brown and Company
Boston   New York   London   Toronto

Nursing Research

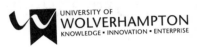

Library of Congress Cataloging-in-Publication Data

Dempsey, Patricia Ann.
　　Nursing research : text and workbook / Patricia Ann Dempsey,
　Arthur D. Dempsey. — 4th ed.
　　　　p.　　cm.
　　Rev. ed. of: Nursing research with basic statistical applications.
　3rd ed. c1992.
　　Includes bibliographical references and index.
　　ISBN 0-316-18188-9
　　1. Nursing—Research.　2. Nursing—Research—Problems, exercises,
　etc.　I. Dempsey, Arthur D.　II. Dempsey, Patricia Ann. Nursing
　research with basic statistical applications.　III. Title.
　　[DNLM:　1. Nursing Research.　WY 20.5 D389n　1996]
　RT81.5.D46　1996
　610.73'072—dc20
　DNLM/DLC
　for Library of Congress　　　　　　　　　　　　　　　　95-40104
　　　　　　　　　　　　　　　　　　　　　　　　　　　　　　CIP

Printed in the United States of America

MV-NY

Editorial: Evan R. Schnittman, Suzanne Jeans
Indexer: Nancy Newman
Production Supervisor: Cate Rickard
Cover Designer: Martucci Studio

For the two Gretchens and the two Helens

Contents

Appendixes   181

Preface

Like the three previous editions of *Nursing Research*, the fourth edition provides basic research principles and techniques for preparation in nursing research at the undergraduate level. The workbook provides application activities that reinforce the material in the text.

The book is carefully designed to guide students through three processes basic to baccalaureate education in nursing research: (1) the research process, (2) the process of critical evaluation of research for scientific merit, and (3) the process of utilizing research in the practice setting.

It continues to be our conviction that students exposed to the research process for the first time find that their learning is facilitated (and their anxiety is reduced) when they are guided through the research process in a systematic manner and provided with activities to reinforce their learning. To enhance the development of essential critiquing skills, step-by-step activities take students through the process of critically evaluating published research studies for scientific merit and applicability to nursing practice. Finally, students are provided with material to understand the issues and the processes involved in utilizing research in the clinical setting. Related practice activities prepare them to begin to participate in research utilization.

Although preparation for writing a research proposal is not usually included in a basic nursing research course at the undergraduate level, Appendix E: Preparing a Research Proposal has been included in the event such information is needed.

P.A.D.
A.D.D.

Acknowledgment

Dr. Judith F. Karshmer, Professor of Nursing at New Mexico State University, deserves special acknowledgment, and our appreciation, for her critical review of the workbook activities and for her contributions to the chapter on research utilization.

Part
1 Becoming Acquainted with Nursing Research

The material in Part I is designed to acquaint you with the nature of research and nursing research. Chapter 1 introduces basic concepts related to the what and why of research in general and nursing research in particular. It also provides a brief overview of the historical development and future trends in nursing research in the United States. Chapter 2 is an overview of the stages of the research process. Chapter 3 presents the traditions of the quantitative and qualitative strategies used by nursing researchers, and Chapter 4 discusses the critical area of ethical behavior that is required of all researchers dealing with human subjects.

1   The Nature of Research and Nursing Research

Objectives

When you have finished reading this chapter you should be able to:

1. Define the term *research*
2. Describe research as a scientific process of inquiry
3. Identify limitations of the scientific research process
4. Classify research activities
5. Describe the nurse's roles in research
6. Explore the historical development of nursing research

What Is Research?
   What Research Is
   What Research Is Not
Research as a Scientific Process of Inquiry
   The Scientific Method
   Order
   Control
   Empiricism
   Generalization
   Purposes of Research
   Research in Nursing
Limitations of the Scientific Research Process
Classification of Research Activities
   Classification by Purpose
   Classification by Approach
Why Nurses Should Learn about Research
Nursing Research over the Years

What Is Research?

Now that you are beginning your experience with research—particularly nursing research—it is important that you understand what research *is* and what research *is not*.

If you are like many other individuals, you probably associate the word *research* with experiments conducted in the laboratory on various animals, or with the discovery of new drugs or treatment methods in medical science. You may also associate research with the scientific experiments being conducted in space during the past several years. In reality, however, the word *research* has many different meanings and broad applications.

What Research Is

There are as many different views of what research is as there are writers who offer such views. We have attempted to synthesize these views and offer the following description of what research is:

> **Research** is a scientific process of inquiry and/or experimentation that involves purposeful, systematic, and rigorous collection of data. Analysis and interpretation of the data are then made in order to gain new knowledge or add to existing knowledge. Research has the ultimate aim of developing an organized body of scientific knowledge.

What Research Is Not

Before we look further at what research is, let us take some time to look at what it is not. Research is not going to the library to collect existing information on a specific topic and then writing a review of the material, such as in a term paper or research project. This activity, involving the reorganization or restatement of knowledge that is already known, is sometimes referred to as *search* rather than *research*. In order to consider a work as "scientific research," we must use present and past knowledge to answer new questions and to add new knowledge to the fund of already existing knowledge. Research activity is intended to find answers to questions or solutions for problems. Communicating knowledge that already exists, therefore, is not considered research activity unless new questions are answered or new problems solved. Research is conducted only after an extensive examination of materials related to the proposed question or problem has been carried out. This examination determines if the answer to the question or problem is available in present knowledge. If correct answers are readily available, there is no need for new research unless the researcher suspects an error or seeks an alternative solution.

Now that we have taken a look at some of the things research is not, let's return to our previous description of what research is. Again, research can be described as a scientific process of inquiry and/or experimentation that involves purposeful, systematic, and rigorous collection of data. Analysis and interpretation of the data are then made in order to gain new knowledge or add to existing knowledge, with the ultimate aim of developing a body of scientific knowledge.

Research as a Scientific Process of Inquiry

Science is a branch of knowledge or study concerned with deriving systematized knowledge by establishing and organizing facts, principles, and methods. The goal of science is to develop theories in order to explain, predict, or control phenomena.

The Scientific Method

In research, the *scientific method,* an orderly process that uses the principles of science, is used. The scientific method requires the use of certain sequential steps to acquire dependable information in solving problems. The scientific method is characterized by (1) order, (2) control, (3) empiricism, and (4) generalization [1].

Order

The scientific approach to problem solving requires the application of *order* and discipline so that confidence in the investigation's results can be assured. This entails the use of the scientific method, in which a series of systematic steps is followed: (1) identification of a problem to be investigated, (2) collection of information according to a previously designed plan (which bears on the solution to the problem), (3) analysis of the information, and (4) formulation of conclusions regarding the problem being investigated.

Control

Control of factors not relevant to the investigation is an essential element of the scientific method. This means that the investigator must try to identify the effects of the factors not directly investigated in connection with the identified problem, and must try to keep them from influencing those factors identified for study. For example, when investigating the relationship between cerebrovascular accidents and the use of oral contraceptives, the investigator must take measures to control such influences as stress, diet, and other factors contributing to the development of atherosclerosis.

Empiricism

The scientific method is also characterized by *empiricism*. That is, the evidence gathered to generate new knowledge must be rooted in objective reality and must be gathered directly or indirectly through the five human senses: sight, sound, smell, taste, and touch.

Generalization

Generalization, another characteristic of the scientific method, means that the investigator does not use the scientific method merely to understand isolated events, but must also be able to apply the investigation's results to a broader setting. For example, in an experimental clinical study designed to investigate the effectiveness of stockinette caps on conservation of body heat in newborn infants, 40 infants from the newborn nursery of a private hospital were sampled in such a way as to ensure that they and their mothers were equivalent and normal subjects (newborn) [2]. The infants were randomly placed in an experimental group (stockinette caps) or a control group (no caps). Temperatures were measured at 5 minutes and 30 minutes after birth. The extent of temperature loss was recorded and the differences in the mean heat loss was reported. The ultimate aim of the study was not merely to analyze the effect of stockinette caps on the specific infants in the study, rather, the study was designed to draw conclusions about the effect that stockinette caps had on newborn infants in general. The kinds of generalizations that result from such research studies assist in the development of scientific theories, thus providing explanations and predictions of future events.

Purposes of Research

Research involves finding answers to questions or solutions to problems, discovering and interpreting new facts, testing theories in order to revise accepted theories or laws in the light of new facts, and formulating new theories. Finally, research has as its ultimate aim the development of an organized body of scientific knowledge that is systematized and that can be useful in explaining, predicting, or controlling phenomena. An example of the usefulness of theory in predicting phenomena is the use of locus of control theory to predict the preoperative coping behavior of children [3].

Research in Nursing

Nursing research is research conducted to answer questions or to find solutions to problems that fall within the specific orientation defined as nursing—that is, "the diagnosis and treatment of human responses to actual or potential health problems" [4]. In complementing biomedical research that focuses primarily on the causes and treatment of disease, nursing research examines "the biological, biomedical and behavioral processes that underlie health and the environment in which health care is delivered" [5]. Nursing research is done to develop an organized body of scientific knowledge that is unique to nursing:

> Nursing research develops knowledge about health and the promotion of health over the full life span, care of persons with health problems and disabilities, and nursing actions to enhance the ability of individuals to respond effectively to actual or potential health problems. . . . Research conducted by nurses includes various types of studies in order to derive clinical interventions to assist those who require nursing care. The complexity of nursing research and its broad scope often require scientific underpinning from several disciplines. Hence, nursing research cuts across traditional research lines and draws its methods from several fields. [6]

The goal of nursing research is twofold. Nursing research adds to nursing's scientific knowledge base and improves the practice of nursing for the ultimate improvement of patient care: "Research-based practice is essential if the nursing profession is to meet its mandate to society for effective and efficient patient care" [7].

Throughout the past several years, nurses conducting research have added to nursing's scientific knowledge base for the improvement of patient care with studies on such topics as the effects of information on postsurgical coping; [8] adherence to health care regimens among elderly women; [9] the effect of medication distribution systems on medication errors; [10] and uncertainty and adjustment during radiotherapy [11].

Limitations of the Scientific Research Process

Although the scientific research process is usually considered the highest form of attaining human knowledge, it has a number of limitations involving the types of problems that can be investigated. Questions involving morality or value systems cannot be explored with the scientific research approach. Questions dealing with complex social and psychological phenomena, such as anger and anxiety, are also very difficult to investigate because of the problems involved in measuring these phenomena. When human subjects are needed in the study, constraints to protect them often cause additional difficulties. Such constraints have even precluded the application of the scientific method to the investigation of certain problems. This crucial consideration is discussed in detail in later chapters.

Classification of Research Activities

If you are going to understand research, it will be helpful to know the meaning of some commonly used research terms used to classify research activities.

Classification by Purpose

Research may be classified by *purpose*—that is, as either *basic research* or *applied research*. This classification reflects the degree to which the findings can be applied to practical problems in the everyday world. *Basic research,* also called *pure research,* is primarily concerned with establishing new knowledge and with the development or refinement of theories. The findings of basic research may not be immediately applicable to practical problems, but they do provide basic scientific knowledge for building further research. Basic research is really "knowledge for the sake of knowledge." This is in contrast to *applied research,* which is also concerned with establishing new knowledge but is further concerned with knowledge that can be applied in practical settings without undue delay. Applied research has been referred to as "practical application of the theoretical." In general, basic research in the behavioral sciences serves to discover general laws concerning human behavior, while applied research generates knowledge about the operation of these laws in specific settings. However, the distinction between basic and applied research often may not be as clear-cut as we have described. Sometimes the results of basic research studies can be applied in a practical setting, while findings from applied research studies can have theoretical implications and may serve as the focus for basic research.

The majority of nursing studies are examples of applied research. For example, the studies conducted by Lindeman and Van Aernam [12], Lindeman [13], and King and Tarsitano [14] on the value of structured preoperative teaching, deep breathing, coughing, and bed exercises have applications in practical settings. Two basic research studies conducted in nursing are McKinnon-Mullette's study [15] concerned with circulation research and its potential in clinical nursing research, and Raff's study [16] of the relationship of planned prenatal exercise to postnatal growth and development in the offspring of albino rats.

Classification by Approach

Research may also be classified by *approach*. There are three major approaches: descriptive, experimental, and historical. The *descriptive research approach* raises questions based on the ongoing events of the present. The *experimental research approach* raises questions based on the need to manipulate specific conditions in a controlled or laboratory-like setting in order to investigate the effects of different conditions. And in the *historical research approach,* researchers investigate questions based on the past by using procedures designed to determine the accuracy of statements or facts about past events. Each of these approaches is discussed in more detail in the chapters in Part II.

Why Nurses Should Learn about Research

One characteristic of a professional group is that it has a unique body of knowledge and skill. It is generally agreed that nursing is still in the process of defining not only what nursing is, but also what constitutes its unique body of knowledge and skill. In view of this, nursing needs to direct its efforts toward systematic investigation of questions related to the practice and profession of nursing.

The 1985 guidelines for nursing research prepared by the American Nurses' Association Cabinet on Nursing Research recognize the essential nature of research in improving nursing practice into the twenty-first century:

> The future of Nursing practice and, ultimately, the future of health care in this country depend on nursing research designed to constantly generate an up-to-date, organized body of nursing knowledge. Society and its approach to health care are experiencing rapid change. . . . Thus, nursing research needs to proceed in orderly directions, generating knowledge built on previous information in order to provide the foundation for nursing education and practice in the twenty-first century. [17]

The 1993 position statement on education for participation in nursing research, prepared by the American Nurses' Association Council of Nurse Researchers, defines elements of competence in research that are appropriate to nurses prepared in different types of nursing education programs at the associate degree, baccalaureate, master's, doctoral, and postdoctoral levels [18].

If nursing is to develop an organized body of scientific knowledge, there are several ways that you as a nurse can participate. First, you must develop the ability to read nursing literature critically as a means of validating nursing practice, discovering gaps in knowledge, and evaluating the findings of research studies. Then you can decide whether or not the knowledge could be used in caring for your patients. This is such an important goal that we have included throughout this text the principles and techniques of critical evaluation. With a basic research orientation, you will also be able to generate hunches and raise questions on the basis of which research studies can be carried out. Finally, you may want to become involved, either as a principal investigator or as a participant, in a research project that will contribute new knowledge.

Although the emphasis on research in nursing has become a relatively strong movement only within the past 30 to 35 years, historically, nursing research has been emerging over a period of more than a hundred years. The next section provides a brief overview of the historical development of aspects of nursing that have significantly affected the development of nursing research.

Nursing Research over the Years

When Florence Nightingale established her system of nursing and nursing education over a hundred years ago, she envisioned the development of a scholarly, humane, and scientific discipline. She utilized the research process and used her detailed records to formulate ideas for improving nursing and health care. She encouraged nurses to develop the habit of sound observation:

> In dwelling upon the vital importance of *sound* observation, it must never be lost sight of what observation is for. It is not for the sake of piling up miscellaneous information or curious facts, but for the sake of saving life and increasing health and comfort. [emphasis in original] [19]

If nursing education in the United States had followed the principles to which Florence Nightingale was dedicated, nursing research might have progressed more swiftly. However, the development of hospital schools of nursing, with their primary emphasis on nursing service by students, resulted in the placement of nurses in subservient roles. Nurses cared primarily for individuals who were ill and meticulously carried out the orders of authority figures, usually physicians. Unfortunately for the progress of nursing research, nurses who accepted these subservient roles were hardly able to develop or refine the questioning attitude and abstract thinking associated with the scientific method of inquiry.

From 1900 to 1950, most leaders in nursing had advanced preparation in the field of education. As a result, many research studies focused on education for nursing rather than the practice of nursing. The majority of these studies were concerned with the characteristics of nursing students themselves as well as with their educational preparation.

Articles in the nursing literature from 1900 to 1950 show nurses concerned and writing about the care of patients with communicable diseases, hygiene and sanitation, asepsis, and high maternal and infant death rates. The first case studies appeared in the *American Journal of Nursing* in the 1920s. They were used as teaching tools for students, as well as patient progress records to improve patient care. By 1930, the need to distinguish nursing orders from medical orders and to evaluate the effectiveness of nursing procedures appeared. Articles began to express the need for student nurses to be free to criticize and to be relieved of excessive nursing service duties in order to benefit fully from their educational programs.

In the late 1940s, after World War II, the broader concept of nursing as practiced by public health nurses became accepted. The primary focus on nursing care for the hospitalized patient was expanded to include the patient and family in a variety of settings, in cooperation with physicians and other health professionals, and the prevention of illness and the promotion of health. An awareness grew of the need for nurses to acquire knowledge of the social, behavioral, and natural sciences, as well as the humanities, in order to care for their patients and their families.

In the 1950s, recognition of the need to prepare nurses at the graduate level for leadership positions, advanced practice, and research contributed to the advancement of nursing research.

In order to communicate the growing body of nursing research, the first issue of *Nursing Research* was published in 1952. *Nursing Research* serves as an important resource devoted to the issues and problems associated with nursing research and to the publication of nursing research studies. In 1955, the American Nurses' Association established the American Nurses' Foundation, which supports and promotes research in nursing.

Nurses writing since the 1950s have reflected ideas about the conceptual development of nursing, nursing as a science, and the educational preparation needed for nurses to conduct research. From 1955 to 1965, researchers focused on student characteristics, selection and retention of students, and the educational process. Articles dealing with the quality of patient care began to appear in the literature. Research studies focused on long-term care and rehabilitation of patients and on problems of patients with chronic diseases such as heart disease, cancer, and strokes. Hospitals began to report experiences with intensive care and automation.

Prior to the 1970s, *Nursing Research* was the only major publication devoted to communicating the results of nursing research studies. Since that time, nursing research reports and articles representing perspectives on the development of nursing as a science have been included in such journals as the *Western Journal of Nursing Research, Research in Nursing and Health, Advances in Nursing Science, Nursing Science Quarterly,* and *Scholarly Inquiry for Nursing Practice.*

In 1970, the National Commission for the Study of Nursing and Nursing Education, funded by the American Nurses' Association and additional private sources, published the findings of its independent investigation of the quality of U.S. nursing [20]. The commission reported that nursing in the United States presented an "impoverished figure" in terms of research capacity and support. At that time, there was very little public or private funding for nursing research. Fewer than 500 U.S. nurses held earned doctoral degrees, the generally accepted level for research competence. Many of these individuals had been prepared for educational administration or teaching, as there were almost no doctoral programs with specific preparation for research into clinical nursing practice or nursing intervention [21]. Thus, little research had been done on the actual effects of nursing intervention and care. Nursing had few definitive guides for the improvement of practice:

> Lack of research leaves us without a body of facts or a set of probabilities to guide or assess the nursing care of a patient. Of necessity, nursing practice today consists of stereotyped techniques sprinkled liberally with personal idiosyncrasy. . . . Since we have not developed valid means for assessing the effects of varied interventions, it is almost impossible to define optimum nursing care. [22]

The 1973 report of the National Commission on Nursing emphasized that nursing was still more an art than a science. Nurse-patient interactions continued to be characterized by a combination of individual judgment, concern for the patient, and supportive care, rather than with procedures based on validated scientific knowledge. However, with the increased amount and complexity of knowledge concerning human health and response to illness, the art of nursing was no longer sufficient to ensure optimum patient care. "The aim of research should be to elevate the practice of nursing—not art *or* science, but art *and* science are needed to ensure the highest levels of humane and capable care" [23] [emphasis in original].

In 1981, Lysaught [24] reported on the extent to which the recommendations of the National Commission for the Study of Nursing and Nursing Education had been implemented over a period of 8 years. The report optimistically predicted that the increase in the number of doctoral programs in nursing since the initiation of the National Commission's study should provide for a greater supply of nurses with "investigative skills for conceptual and theoretical inquiry into nursing that will extend the scientific base of all nursing practice" [25]. The report also pointed out that in the area of federal funding for nursing research, there had been a "dramatic increase" that had been generally related to the levels recommended in the 1970 report of the National Commission. These funds, however, "have often been used as pawns in political maneuvering, and the result is that planning and execution of research have often suffered through the vagaries of administrative and legislative battling" [26].

An analysis of publications related to nursing practice research reflects, to some extent, the degree to which the recommendations and predictions of the National Commission have been realized. Moody and colleagues analyzed 720 journal articles published in the decade between 1977 and 1986 that reported results of nursing practice research. Findings showed that 95 percent of research in nursing practice reported during this time was conducted by nurses as first authors, over half of them with doctoral degrees. One-third of the studies focused on nursing intervention, and two-thirds focused on assessment. These published studies also reflected an increase in research funding during this decade [27].

In 1976 and 1981, and again in 1985, the American Nurses' Association developed a statement of priorities for research in nursing, designed to guide nurse researchers in the study of areas of nursing that are crucial to the scientific advancement of the nursing profession. The 1985 Priorities for Nursing Research, developed by the ANA Cabinet on Nursing Research, are listed in Chapter 5 of this text.

With the establishment of the National Center for Nursing Research (NCNR) in 1986, nursing research made a dramatic advance into the mainstream of health care science. Dr. Ada Sue Hinshaw summarized this historical milestone for nursing in remarks at her swearing-in ceremony as its first director:

> The establishment of the National Center for Nursing Research (NCNR) on April 18, 1986, by Secretary Bowen was an historic moment for the nursing profession. It provides a focal point from which to stimulate and facilitate the generation and testing of scientific knowledge to guide the practice of one of the country's largest health care professions. . . . The National Center's union with the National Institutes of Health is particularly significant for it brings nursing research into the mainstream of health care science. It allows for nursing research to be developed/conducted in collaboration with the other scientific disciplines in a complementary manner. . . . In turn, knowledge from nursing research can and will be incorporated in the broader base of health care science as a result of being developed and tested within this collaborative interdisciplinary environment. [28]

In 1993, the National Center for Nursing Research became the National Institute of Nursing Research (NINR) within the National Institutes of Health.

Currently, there have been major expansions in research related to clinical practice, growing concerns about ethical practices, and the protection of human subjects. Nurses are increasingly studying *nursing*. They see an urgent need to investigate the organization and delivery of nursing care to patients. Predictions for the direction of nursing research, for the remainder of this century and into the twenty-first century, indicate an increased concentration on research designed to investigate clinical nursing practice in all settings, continued evolution of nursing theories, more organizational activities to increase the utilization of research results in practice, and significant progress toward the ultimate goal of extending the scientific basis for nursing in order to improve the delivery of patient care.

In this chapter we introduced you to some basic concepts related to research and nursing research. In addition we provided a brief overview of the historical development and future of the nursing research movement in the United States.

The Workbook Activities for Chapter 1 will help you apply this information.

References

1. Polit, D., and B. Hungler. 1995. *Nursing Research: Principles and Methods,* 5th ed. Philadelphia: J. B. Lippincott, pp. 9–10.
2. Klingner, S. J. 1992. "The Effect of Stockinette Caps on Conservation of Body Heat in Newborn Infants." In P. Dempsey and A. Dempsey. *Nursing Research with Basic Statistical Applications.* Boston: Jones and Bartlett, pp. 227–243.
3. LaMontagne, Lynda L. 1984. "Children's Locus of Control Beliefs as Predictors of Preoperative Coping Behavior." *Nursing Research,* 33 (March–April): 76–79.
4. American Nurses' Association. 1980. *Nursing: A Social Policy Statement.* Kansas City: American Nurses' Association, p. 3.
5. National Center for Nursing Research. 1987. *Nursing Science: Serving Health through Research,* October. Bethesda, MD: National Institutes of Health.
6. American Nurses' Association Commission on Nursing Research. 1981. *Research Priorities for the 1980s: Generating a Scientific Basis for Nursing Practice.* Code No. D-68 2M. Kansas City: American Nurses' Association.
7. American Nurses' Association. 1993. *Position Statement on Education for Participation in Nursing Research.* Washington, D.C.: American Nurses' Association, p. 1.
8. Ziemer, M. 1983. "The Effects of Information on Postsurgical Coping." *Nursing Research,* 32: 282–287.
9. Chang, B., et al. 1985. "Adherence to Health Care Regimens among Elderly Women." *Nursing Research,* 34: 27–31.
10. Long, G. 1982. "The Effect of Medication Distribution Systems on Medication Errors." *Nursing Research,* 31 (May–June): 182–184.
11. Christman, N. J. 1990. "Uncertainty and Adjustment During Radiotherapy." *Nursing Research,* 39 (January–February): 17–20.
12. Lindeman, C. A., and B. Van Aernam. 1971. "Nursing Intervention

with the Presurgical Patient—The Effects of Structured and Unstructured Preoperative Teaching." *Nursing Research,* 20 (July–August): 319–332.

13. Lindeman, C. A. 1972. "Nursing Intervention with the Presurgical Patient: Effectiveness and Efficiency of Group and Individual Preoperative Teaching—Phase Two." *Nursing Research,* 21 (May–June): 196–209.

14. King, I., and B. Tarsitano. 1982. "The Effect of Structured and Unstructured Preoperative Teaching: A Replication." *Nursing Research,* 31 (November–December): 324–329.

15. McKinnon-Mullette, E. 1972. "Approaches to the Study of Nursing Questions and the Development of Nursing Science. Circulation Research: Exploring Its Potential in Clinical Nursing Research." *Nursing Research,* 21 (November-December): 494–498.

16. Raff, B. S. 1977. "The Relationship of Planned Prenatal Exercise to Postnatal Growth and Development in the Offspring of Albino Rats." In F. S. Downs and M. A. Newman, Eds., *A Sourcebook of Nursing Research.* Philadelphia: F. A. Davis, pp. 78–85.

17. American Nurses' Association Cabinet on Nursing Research. 1985. *Directions for Nursing Research: Toward the Twenty-first Century.* Kansas City: American Nurses' Association, p. 1.

18. Ibid. pp. 1–3.

19. Nightingale, F. 1859. *Notes on Nursing.* Philadelphia: J. B. Lippincott, p. 70.

20. National Commission for the Study of Nursing and Nursing Education. 1970. *An Abstract for Action.* New York: McGraw-Hill.

21. Lysaught, J. 1981. *Action in Affirmation: Toward an Unambiguous Profession of Nursing.* New York: McGraw-Hill, p. 59.

22. National Commission for the Study of Nursing, *An Abstract for Action,* p. 84.

23. National Commission for the Study of Nursing and Nursing Education. 1973. *From Abstract into Action.* New York: McGraw-Hill, p. 125.

24. Lysaught, J. 1981. *Action in Affirmation: Toward an Unambiguous Profession of Nursing.* New York: McGraw-Hill.

25. Ibid., p. 64.

26. Ibid., p. 63.

27. Moody, L. E., M. E. Wilson, K. Smyth, R. Schwartz, M. Tittle, and M. L. Van Cott. 1988. "Analysis of a Decade of Nursing Practice Research: 1977–1986." *Nursing Research,* 37 (November–December): 374–379.

28. American Association of Colleges of Nursing. 1987. *AACN Newsletter* (Lester Kip, Ed.), 13 (July): 1.

Bibliography and Suggested Readings

American Association of Colleges of Nursing. 1987. *AACN Newsletter* (Lester Kip, Ed.), 13 (July): 1.

American Nurses' Association. 1980. *Nursing: A Social Policy Statement.* Code No. NP-63 25M 9/83R. Kansas City: American Nurses' Association.

American Nurses' Association Cabinet on Nursing Research. 1985. *Directions for Nursing Research: Toward the Twenty-first Century.* Kansas City: American Nurses' Association.

———. 1993. *Position Statement on Education for Participation in Nursing Research.* Washington, D.C.: American Nurses' Association.

———. 1981. *Research Priorities for the 1980s: Generating a Scientific Basis for Nursing Practice.* Code No. D-68 2M. Kansas City: American Nurses' Association.

Chang, Betty L., Gwen C. Uman, Lawrence S. Linn, John E. Ware, and Robert L. Kane. 1985. "Adherence to Health Care Regimens among Elderly Women." *Nursing Research,* 34: 27–31.

Christman, N. J. 1990. "Uncertainty and Adjustment During Radiotherapy." *Nursing Research,* 39 (January–February): 17–20.

Dempsey, P., and A. Dempsey. 1992. *Nursing Research with Basic Statistical Applications.* Boston: Jones and Bartlett.

Dempsey, P., and T. Gesse. 1983. "The Childbearing Haitian Refugee—Cultural Applications to Clinical Nursing." *Public Health Reports,* 98 (May–June): 261–267.

———. 1985. "The Childbearing Cuban Refugee: A Cultural Profile." *Urban Health,* 14 (May): 32–37.

Dempsey, P., and P. Hippo. 1990. "Beliefs and Practices of Spanish Speaking Childbearing Women from Mexico." Unpublished manuscript.

Downs, F. S., and M. A. Newman. 1977. *A Sourcebook of Nursing Research.* Philadelphia: F. A. Davis.

Fawcett, J. 1984. "Hallmarks of Success in Nursing Research." *Advances in Nursing Science,* 7 (October): 1–11.

———. 1986. "A Typology of Nursing Research Activities According to Educational Preparation." *Journal of Professional Nursing,* 1: 75–78.

Fitzpatrick, J. J. 1988. "How Can We Enhance Nursing Knowledge and Nursing Practice?" *Nursing and Health Care,* 9 (November/December): 516–521.

Gortner, S. 1980. "Generating a Scientific Basis for Nursing Practice: Research Priorities for the 1980s." *Nursing Research,* 29 (July–August): 219.

———. 1983. "The History and Philosophy of Nursing Science and Research." *Advances in Nursing Science,* 5 (January): 1–8.

Gortner, S., and H. Nahm. 1977. "An Overview of Nursing Research in the United States." *Nursing Research,* 26 (January–February): 10–30.

Hopkins, C. D. 1976. *Educational Research: A Structure for Inquiry.* Columbus, OH: Charles E. Merrill.

King, I., and B. Tarsitano. 1982. "The Effect of Structured and Unstructured Preoperative Teaching: A Replication." *Nursing Research,* 31 (November–December): 324–329.

Klingner, Sarah J. 1992. "The Effect of Stockinette Caps on Conservation of Body Heat in Newborn Infants." In P. Dempsey and A. Dempsey, *Nursing Research with Basic Statistical Applications.* Boston: Jones and Bartlett. pp. 227–243.

LaMontagne, Lynda L. 1984. "Children's Locus of Control Beliefs as Predictors of Preoperative Coping Behavior." *Nursing Research,* 33 (March–April): 76–79, 85.

Lindeman, C. A. 1972. "Nursing Intervention with the Pre-surgical Patient: Effectiveness and Efficiency of Group and Individual Preoperative Teaching—Phase Two." *Nursing Research,* 21 (May–June): 196–209.

———. 1973. "Nursing Research: A Visible, Viable Component of Nursing Practice." *Journal of Nursing Administration,* 3 (March–April): 18–21.

Lindeman, C. A., and B. Van Aernam. 1971. "Nursing Intervention with the Presurgical Patient—The Effects of Structured and Unstructured Preoperative Teaching." *Nursing Research,* 20 (July–August): 319–332.

Long, G. 1982. "The Effect of Medication Distribution Systems on Medication Errors." *Nursing Research,* 31 (May–June): 182–184.

Lysaught, J. 1981. *Action in Affirmation: Toward an Unambiguous Profession of Nursing.* New York: McGraw-Hill.

McKinnon-Mullette, E. 1972. "Approaches to the Study of Nursing Questions and the Development of Nursing Science: Circulation Research: Exploring Its Potential in Clinical Nursing Research." *Nursing Research,* 21 (November–December): 494–498.

McMurrey, P. H. 1982. "Toward a Unique Knowledge Base in Nursing." *Image,* 14: 86–88.

Moody, L. E., M. E. Wilson, K. Smyth, R. Schwartz, M. Tittle, and M. L. Van Cott. 1988. "Analysis of a Decade of Nursing Practice Research: 1977–1986." *Nursing Research,* 37 (November–December): 374–379.

National Center for Nursing Research. 1987. *Nursing Science: Serving Health through Research,* October. Bethesda, MD: National Institutes of Health.

National Commission for the Study of Nursing and Nursing Education. 1970. *An Abstract for Action.* New York: McGraw-Hill.

———. 1973. *From Abstract into Action.* New York: McGraw-Hill.

Nightingale, F. 1859. *Notes on Nursing.* Philadelphia: J. B. Lippincott.

Peplau, H. E. 1988. "The Art and Science of Nursing." *Nursing Science Quarterly* 1 (February): 8–15.

Polit, D., and B. Hungler. 1995. *Nursing Research: Principles and Methods,* 5th ed. Philadelphia: J. B. Lippincott.

Raff, B. S. 1977. "The Relationship of Planned Prenatal Exercise to Postnatal Growth and Development in the Offspring of Albino Rats." In F. S. Downs and M. A. Newman, Eds., *A Sourcebook of Nursing Research,* 2nd ed. Philadelphia: F. A. Davis, pp. 78–85.

Wysocki, A. B. 1983. "Basic vs. Applied Research." *Western Journal of Nursing Research,* 5: 217–224.

Ziemer, M. 1983. "The Effects of Information on Postsurgical Coping." *Nursing Research,* 32: 282–287.

2 Stages of the Research Process

Objectives

When you have finished reading this chapter you should be able to:

1. Identify research as a process for scientific inquiry
2. List the steps of the research process
3. Identify the steps of the research process as stages in the process of scientific inquiry
4. Compare the research process with the problem-solving process

---

Overview of the Research Process
Stages of the Research Process
    Stage I: Planning the Study
    Stage II: Implementing the Research Proposal
    Stage III: Communicating the Results of the Study
Relationship of the Research Process to the Problem-Solving
    Process
    Comparison between Research and Problem Solving
    Which Approach Is "Better"?
Summary

In Chapter 1 we discussed the nature of research in general and nursing research in particular. Chapter 2 will acquaint you with the nature of the research process and its relationship to the problem-solving process. It describes the three stages of the research process that are used in conducting a research study.

Overview of the Research Process

As you become acquainted with research terminology, you will see the term *research process* used to refer to the systematic steps, or ongoing phases, involved in conducting a research study. Although the number and order of these steps may vary, the following list contains those commonly used:

1. Statement of the research problem
2. Review of related literature
3. Statement of the purpose of the study
4. Collection of data
5. Analysis and interpretation of data
6. Formulation of conclusions and implications
7. Communication of the results of the study

Remember, conducting a study using the research process is a systematic, planned activity that can be thought of as a chain of reasoning. It begins with a statement of the problem and proceeds systematically to the communication of the study's results: "The total process from problem isolation to the addition of new knowledge is a logically structured inquiry into some well-defined problem" [1].

Stages of the Research Process

It is helpful to consider the systematic steps of the research process as consisting of three sequential stages that should answer the research question or solve the research problem: (1) planning, (2) implementation, and (3) communication.

Stage I: Planning the Study

The initial stage of the research process is the planning stage. Here the problem question, which the research will answer, is selected and refined into a problem statement, and the methodology for the study is formulated. The problem must be researchable and the answer not already known. The research should contribute to new knowledge. Appropriate methods must be available to investigate the problem. Consideration must be given to the availability of subjects expected to participate in the study, as well as to the ethical implications of the research, such as the protection of the study participants' rights. The constraints of time and money imposed by the study are also important considerations in selecting the problems to be studied. Examples of general problem areas in nursing might include preoperative teaching of hysterectomy patients, compliance of diabetic patients with prescribed treatment regimens, and family caregivers' ways of coping with the home-bound elderly.

To place the problem in the context of what is already known, the researcher then reviews the literature related to the problem, citing references to significant publications and journal articles pertaining to that problem. Because the objective of nursing research is to contribute to scientific knowledge, the problem may be placed within a theory or based on concepts to which the study's results can be related. The literature review summarizes existing knowledge in relation to the problem and helps the investigator to learn more about the problem area. Next, the researcher may use the information gained so far to predict the outcome of the study. This is done by formulating a *hypothesis*—an educated guess—that will be used to guide the rest of the study. Testing the hypothesis then becomes the purpose for conducting the study. Not all research studies are conducted to test hypotheses; some studies are designed to answer questions or describe phenomena.

All of the terms relating to the study must be carefully defined so there will be no question about what the researcher means when using the terms.

The methodology for the study defines the way pertinent information will be gathered in order to answer the research question or analyze the research problem. This includes detailed discussion on the selection of subjects who will participate in the study, and description of the data collection procedures and techniques. Also included is a plan for analyzing the data after they have been collected in a form that facilitates analysis. Limitations of the study are included to identify particular aspects of the study over which the researcher has no control.

Thus, the planning stage of the research process consists of the first five steps in the research process: (1) statement of the problem, (2) review of related literature, (3) statement of the purpose of the study, (4) plans for collection of the data, and (5) plans for analysis of the data.

In order to structure the planning stage of a research study, the researcher formulates a *research proposal:* a detailed written description of the proposed study. Sometimes called a prospectus, the research proposal serves as a blueprint for the research project and *must* be completed *before* conducting either a quantitative or a qualitative research study. The written proposal communicates the problem being investigated and the procedures that will be used in the investigation.

A research proposal is written for several purposes. Having to sit down and write a proposal for the research study forces the researcher to think through various aspects of the study that might not otherwise have been considered. The plan can then be evaluated by others, who may improve it by suggesting something that has been left out or by considering whether or not the ideas would be workable in the actual study setting. The written proposal provides a step-by-step guide to follow in carrying out the research project. It saves the researcher from having to remember the many details already considered and the anticipated problems already solved. A well-thought-out proposal saves time, helps avoid mistakes, and should result in a higher quality research study. Written research proposals are required for all academic research studies, such as theses and dissertations, and for all research submitted for funding by various government agencies and private organizations.

In developing a research proposal (step 1 of the planning stage of the research process), information related to the first five steps of the research process is included. It is generally agreed that the information to be reviewed here should be included in a research proposal. Each of these components will be discussed in more detail in subsequent chapters. Step-by-step guidelines for the development of a research proposal are included in Appendix E.

1. *Statement of the problem:* This section should include the background of the problem and a brief statement of what is being investigated. The significance of the study should also be stated.
2. *Review of related literature:* This section presents summaries of other studies and articles that are related to the problem. It may also include the concepts or theory on which the research is based.
3. *Statement of the purpose of the study:* This section contains a clear statement of the purpose for conducting the research. It may be stated as a hypothesis to be tested, a question to be answered, or a phenomenon to be described or analyzed.
4. *Definitions of the terms used in the study*
5. *Plan for data collection:* This section should include detailed descriptions of the study subjects to be selected, and should describe the data collection techniques and procedures. Assumptions and limitations of the study may also be included here.
6. *Plan for data analysis:* This section contains procedures for analyzing the study data, including the kinds of tables to be used. If you plan to carry out a study requiring the use of statistics but do not have a statistical background, you will need help with this section of the proposal.
7. *Bibliography*
8. *Appendixes* (optional): This section may include materials developed especially for the study (cover letters, consent forms, questionnaires, interview schedules, and so forth).

Stage II: Implementing the Research Proposal

After the completed research proposal has been evaluated by those who can offer suggestions and, perhaps, revised to incorporate their suggestions, it must be approved by the appropriate institutional committees. This is very important, for it assures the protection of the rights of the study subjects as well as conformity to the policies and procedures of the institution. Once this approval is given, the researcher is then ready to implement the written proposal. It is in the implementation stage of the research process that the actual collection and analysis of data for the research study take place. In this stage, the researcher follows the written proposal by systematically gathering data for analysis. If unexpected problems arise in the research situation, the researcher may decide to alter the procedures while still implementing the written proposal as closely as possible.

Stage III: Communicating the Results of the Study

After analyzing the data in relation to the research problem, the researcher formulates conclusions, discusses them, and relates these conclusions to relevant present knowledge. The researcher should cite implications of the research and formulate recommendations for further study. The researcher then writes a report of the complete study to communicate its findings so that others have access to the knowledge. Research reports vary from formal reports to abridged reports for publication. A formal research report usually contains the following information and will be discussed further in Chapter 11.

The research report is divided into three major parts: (1) preliminary materials, (2) main body (text) of the report, and (3) reference materials. Each main part consists of several sections, as follows:

1. *Preliminary materials:* The preliminary section includes the title page, table of contents, list of illustrations or figures, list of tables, an abstract, and a preface or acknowledgment, if any.
2. *Main body* (text) of the report:
    a. The *introduction* includes the statement of the problem, a review of related literature, the conceptual or theoretical framework, the purposes of the study, and a definition of terms.
    b. *Methodology* includes the research approach, a description of the study subjects, the techniques used for data collection, the procedures, the assumptions, and the limitations of the study.
    c. The *findings* include the presentation of the data that have been collected for the study.
    d. The *discussion* includes interpretation of the findings by the investigator, implications for nursing, and recommendations for further study.
    e. The *summary* includes a brief restatement of the problem, purpose, major findings, conclusions, and recommendations.
3. *Reference materials:* This section includes the bibliography and appendixes.

Comparing these components of the research report with those of a research proposal, you will see that the completed research report has the added components of data analysis and interpretation, as well as conclusions and recommendations for further study. This is logical when you recall that the proposal is written in the planning stage of the research process and describes what the researcher proposes to do. The completed research report represents the implementation stage and describes what the researcher actually did and found.

Because the research proposal is written in the future tense, much of its content may be used in writing the research report by changing the tense from future to past.

The ultimate aim of conducting research into the practice and profession of nursing and communicating the results is to use the knowledge for the improvement of patient care and of the nursing profession. Nursing research has become a valued activity as nursing strives to identify and construct its scientific knowledge base. But there is a time lag between the reporting of nursing research knowledge and its utilization in practice. Although nurses are expected to know the research that has been conducted and to use the findings as a basis for scientific practice, the majority of nurses are not prepared to read research journals critically and do not attend research conferences. Thus, *research utilization* may be more practically viewed "as an organizational process to be carried out by and for the total staff in a department of nursing" [2].

Research utilization is discussed further in Chapter 12.

Relationship of the Research Process to the Problem-Solving Process

Even though research and problem solving are often compared, it is important to understand that the research process and the problem-solving process are not the same. The two processes differ in their purpose. Problem solving is a simpler process: Its purpose is to find an immediate solution to a practical problem in an actual setting. The basic purpose of research, on the other hand, goes beyond solving the immediate problem: It provides new knowledge that can be generalized to a broader setting and can be used to benefit a larger number of people. For example, the nurse may decide that the application of a stockinette cap to a newborn infant would be an effective way to conserve body heat (problem solving). In contrast, a systematic research study (such as the study discussed in Chap. 1), conducted in relation to the same patient care problem, would be expected to benefit a large number of patients (provided that the design of the study permits its results to be generalized).

Table 2-1. Comparison of the Stages of the Research Process with the Problem-Solving Process

Stage	Research Process	Problem-Solving Process
Planning	Written proposal includes specific problem statement; literature review to place research problem within existing knowledge and within theoretical or conceptual framework if indicated; precise statement of purpose of study; definition of terms; detailed plan for collection and analysis of data.	Detailed written plan not indicated.
Implementation	Institutional assurance of rights of study subjects and conformity to institutional requirements; systematic collection of data according to written proposal; detailed data analysis with appropriate descriptive and inferential statistical technique used.	No formal institutional review indicated. Data collection procedures may not be as rigorous. Simple analytical, statistical, or other method used.
Communication	Written findings should be published so others have access to the new knowledge. Report should be detailed enough to permit replication of the study.	Results and recommendations may be shared with persons in immediate setting.

Comparison between Research and Problem Solving

Table 2-1 compares the research process with the problem-solving process and summarizes the stages of the research process.

Which Approach Is "Better"?

Once you understand that the research process and the problem-solving process have different purposes, it follows that the use of one process rather than the other to investigate a problem should not be considered better or more valuable. The value lies in correctly using the process that is most appropriate for the investigation.

Summary

In this chapter, we considered the nature and components of the research process and its relation to the problem-solving process. The research process was presented as comprising three sequential stages: (1) the planning stage, in which a research proposal is written to describe the study problem and methodology; (2) the implementation stage, in which the completed research proposal is implemented to collect and analyze the data, and (3) the communication stage, in which the researcher formulates conclusions and implications for the study, and writes the report of the study in order to communicate the new knowledge. In order to apply the principles presented, you should complete the Workbook Activities for Chapter 2.

References

1. Hopkins, Charles D. 1976. *Educational Research: A Structure for Inquiry.* Columbus: Charles E. Merrill, p. 13.
2. Horsley, J. A., et al. 1983. *Using Research to Improve Nursing Practice: A Guide.* New York: Grune and Stratton, p. 2.

Bibliography and Selected Readings

Brink, P. J., and M. Wood. 1983. *Basic Steps in Planning Nursing Research.* Belmont, CA: Wadsworth.

———. 1988. *Basic Steps in Planning Nursing Research,* 3rd ed. Boston: Jones and Bartlett.

Fox, D. J. 1982. *Fundamentals of Research in Nursing,* 4th ed. Norwalk, CT: Appleton-Century-Crofts.

Hopkins, C. D. 1976. *Educational Research: A Structure for Inquiry.* Columbus, OH: Charles E. Merrill.

Horsley, J. A., J. Crane, M. K. Crabtree, and D. J. Wood. 1983. *Using Research to Improve Nursing Practice: A Guide.* New York: Grune and Stratton.

Kidder, L. H., C. M. Judd, and E. R. Smith. 1986. *Research Methods in Social Relations,* 5th ed. New York; Holt, Rinehart and Winston.

Polit, D., and B. Hungler. 1987. *Nursing Research: Principles and Methods,* 3rd ed. Philadelphia: J. B. Lippincott.

Van Dalen, D. B. 1973. *Understanding Educational Research.* New York: McGraw-Hill.

Wandelt, Mabel. 1970. *Guide for the Beginning Researcher.* New York: Appleton-Century-Crofts.

3   The Quantitative and Qualitative Traditions of Inquiry

Objectives

When you have finished reading this chapter you should be able to:

1. Discuss the differences between quantitative and qualitative research

2. Define the following terms: numerical analysis, control, and replication

3. Characterize basic qualitative methods

The Nature of Quantitative and Qualitative Methodology
Quantitative Research
Qualitative Research
Qualitative Research Strategies
    Phenomenology
    Ethnography
    Grounded Theory
Summary

The material in this chapter will introduce you to two major traditions of scientific inquiry—the quantitative approach and the qualitative approach—and to the use of each approach in investigating nursing problems.

The Nature of Quantitative and Qualitative Methodology

Traditionally, the scientific method of inquiry has been equated with the use of *quantitative research methods* to investigate the variables selected for study. (A *variable* is something that can have more than one value. Height, weight, hair color, and blood pressure all could be variables.) In quantitative research, the variables are preselected and defined by the investigator, and the data are collected and quantified—translated into numbers—and statistically analyzed with a view to establishing cause-and-effect relationships among the variables. The quantitative approach to research has its roots in the tradition of the "hard" or mathematically based sciences and reflects the rigor of the scientific research approach most often associated with such fields as physics and chemistry. The use of quantitative methodology for investigating human behavior has been associated most often with the disciplines of psychology and sociology.

In the *qualitative research method,* the investigator seeks to identify the qualitative (nonnumerical) aspects of the phenomenon under study from the subjects' viewpoint in order to interpret the totality of the phenomenon. "The qualitative type of research refers to the methods and techniques of observing, documenting, analyzing and interpreting attributes, patterns, characteristics, and meanings of specific, contextual or gestaltic features of phenomena under study" [1].

Qualitative research is often considered "soft" because it does not deal with precise numbers and does not have the apparent "objective reality" that is characteristic of the quantitative approach. The qualitative approach has been associated with the social sciences and humanities, primarily the fields of history and philosophy. The use of qualitative methodology for investigating human behavior is frequently associated with the discipline of social anthropology.

Until recently, the quantitative methodologies for scientific research have been the only methods legitimized by the scientific community. "Even when these methods have failed to be as valid and reliable in nursing and other human sciences as they have been in the natural sciences, researchers in nursing have clung to them, feeling that their only claim to the title of scientist lay in the quantitative methods" [2]. There is no doubt that the quantitative methods used in nursing research have resulted in significant contributions to understanding many of the phenomena of nursing. A growing number of nurse researchers, however, in their conviction that the traditional scientific method imposes constraints on the study of humans, are using qualitative methodologies in their belief that "the [scientific] method's inherent nature . . . reduces the human being under study to an object with many small quantitative units . . . [and] gives no clue as to how to fit these small units back into the dynamic whole that is the living human being with whom the nurse interacts in practice" [3].

Quantitative Research

Quantitative research methodology rests on the basic assumption that all of the traits or characteristics that make up the units of both human and nonhuman organisms, as well as nonliving objects, exist in some degree and can be measured objectively. In some cases there is no trace of the trait or characteristic; in other cases there is a small trace of the characteristic; in still other cases, there is a moderate amount of the characteristic. Finally, in some cases there is a great deal of the characteristic present. Since terms like *small, moderate,* and *great deal* are too scientifically imprecise to be particularly useful in the quantification of data, the quantitative scientist must establish a numerical scale in order to determine the amount of the trait or characteristic that is present. For example, a researcher wishing to measure the amount of nicotine in an individual's blood serum might draw a sample of blood and subject the blood to analysis. There should be no nicotine in the blood of a nonsmoker; this level can be called the zero level. As the presence of nicotine is measured in moderate and heavy smokers, the researcher would then be able to establish a strict numerical scale that would quantify the amount of nicotine in the blood.

Similarly, the blood alcohol tests used by law enforcement agencies provide numerical methods for determining if an individual is intoxicated as defined by the laws of a state. A more positive example of such measuring scales is the numerical measurement of blood sugar in individuals to determine if they suffer from diabetes. This information can be used to enhance the quality of life of individuals suffering from diabetes, and continued testing allows such persons to prolong their lives by stabilizing their blood sugar and insulin levels.

Using numerical scales allows the researcher to be "objective" about the research that is being carried out. Such objectivity allows the researcher to be "outside" of the research; that is, the researcher is not emotionally involved with the subject(s) of the research and is unbiased in the interpretation of the results.

Because nursing research deals with humans, it is often difficult for the researcher to remain emotionally uninvolved with the subjects. Measuring physiologic changes in patients as a result of an experimental technique often can provide such objective data. For example, Callow and Pieper found that a 30-degree backrest elevation had no significant impact on the central venous pressure of children who had had cardiac surgery when compared to the central venous pressure taken while the children were in a supine position [4]. Callow and Pieper concluded that this elevation might enhance the children's comfort and safety.

The quantitative method requires that the problem statement and the design of the research be quite specific and detailed prior to conducting the investigation. Attention is paid to identifying factors not being investigated directly in the study and attempting to control their influence on the outcome of the study. Because of the need for control, quantitative researchers often establish a "context-free" environment. The research then takes place in a laboratory or other setting that gives each subject an equal opportunity to be assessed when measured by the data-gathering instrument.

As discussed in Chapter 1, one of the characteristics of the scientific method is generalization. Much quantitative research is designed and conducted with the purpose of predicting from the sample(s) measured to the whole population from which the sample was drawn. This requires that the design of the study and statistical analysis of the data conform to the strict requirements for generalization, which will be discussed later in this book.

The quantitative researcher also wants to understand the how and why of events and may seek to establish cause-and-effect relationships between the study variables. The structure of the process becomes an *if . . . then* statement: If *x* (*the independent variable*) happens, then *y* (*the dependent variable*) will happen. For example, *if* a person is a heavy cigarette smoker (*x*), *then* can we predict that this individual has a higher risk of developing lung cancer (*y*) than a person who is not a heavy cigarette smoker? If this is indeed a cause-and-effect relationship, lung cancer should then be controlled by stopping or significantly reducing smoking behavior. The determination of cause-and-effect relationships among study variables requires manipulation of the variables through experimentation, with careful attention to control of *confounding variables* (variables that may interfere with the direct causal relationship between independent and dependent variables) and *extraneous variables* (variables that are uncontrolled and outside the purpose of the study, which might influence the study's results). These ideas are discussed in greater detail in Chapter 9.

Although experimentation is a characteristic of quantitative research, quantitative research is not limited only to experimentation. Precisely defined and developed data collection instruments can be used to measure predefined variables. These include questionnaires, surveys, structured interviews, and other data-gathering instruments.

A major concern of quantitative researchers is replicability or reproducibility. When a researcher obtains certain results, can another researcher use the same procedures and obtain the same or similar results? True quantitative research demands that the research be able to be replicated by other researchers and that such replication will yield the same or very similar results. Achieving this replication can be extremely difficult when the researcher is investigating the complex world of human behavior.

Qualitative Research

Qualitative research has several distinct characteristics that can be contrasted with quantitative methods. Whereas quantitative researchers generally have only minimal contact with the subjects of the study, qualitative researchers frequently use themselves as the data-gathering instrument.

Rather than using precisely developed data-gathering tools and instruments to gather data about their subjects' knowledge, interests, and backgrounds, many qualitative researchers spend long periods of time with the study's subjects, observing their behaviors and interactions. The researcher keeps detailed notes about the events that have been observed, the interviews that have been carried out, and any other salient facts that might have a bearing on the purpose of the study. Because of the nature of qualitative research, the investigator gathers data in the setting where the activities are taking place.

Because of the mass of data that can be gathered, the qualitative researcher often deals with only a few members of the group being studied. This allows the researcher to focus intently on the subjects and to gather a great deal of information, which must be analyzed very carefully. For example, if a researcher is interested in the activities of student nurses as they learn and practice appropriate patient care, much of the research would take place in a clinical setting. The questions that students ask each other, as well as the questions asked by and of instructors, staff nurses, supervisors, physicians, patients, and any other individuals in the setting, would all be a part of the data gathered by the researcher. In addition to verbal interactions, which the researcher should transcribe if at all possible, nonverbal cues would also be noted. As the study of proxemics has demonstrated, much information can be gathered from a person's posture or stance.

While gathering data, the researcher must attempt to suspend value judgments. This can be difficult if activities are taking place that the researcher considers objectionable. Qualitative researchers can experience feelings of conflict on this point because their nonintervention may be considered a positive acceptance of the subjects' activity. Clearly, in the hospital study mentioned earlier, the researcher would have to intervene if a nursing student was about to make a mistake in patient care that would endanger the patient's well-being.

In planning their research, qualitative researchers often use essentially the same systematic series of steps in their research as quantitative researchers use. The statement of the problem may not be as rigorously defined as in quantitative research, but few qualitative researchers go into the study setting without some notion of the general area they plan to investigate. Qualitative researchers also establish a plan for the process of data collection. Because qualitative researchers are often their own data-collecting instrument, the data collection plan may include only the development and use of field notes. With the data collection devices available today, however, qualitative researchers may also choose to use such instruments as tape recorders and videotapes.

Qualitative researchers also establish a plan to analyze the data and formulate conclusions concerning the data collected. Because the data are qualitative rather than quantitative (numerical), the data analysis method usually does not depend on statistical tests.

Control (the elimination or reduction of confounding or extraneous variables) is difficult but not impossible to achieve. Qualitative researchers can use several methods to ensure that control is provided. The first is the use of multiple informants. If an investigator uses only one informant concerning certain activities, that informant may not really know about the activities under investigation or may choose to be deceptive concerning the activities. Multiple informants reduce the chances of this loss of control. Second, careful rechecking of the researcher's data is essential. Researchers must be careful to report accurately and completely on the data they have gathered and to gather enough data to warrant the conclusions that are formulated.

As we have seen, the scientific method depends on empiricism—the evidence gathered to gain new knowledge must be rooted in objective reality and gathered through the use of the human senses. The root source of knowledge in qualitative research can be described as "cultural (ethnography), social, environmental, and philosophical phenomena to obtain patterned human interactions, symbols, values, world views, historical and general ethnographic lifeways" [5].

Generalization, the ability to use the findings of research on a sample to anticipate the actions of larger populations, is a major goal of scientific inquiry. Because the primary purpose of qualitative research is to elicit meaning, qualitiative researchers are often unable to generalize from their findings to larger populations. "Remember, generalizability is not the purpose of qualitative research but the purpose is rather to elicit meaning in a given situation and to develop reality-based theory" [6]. However, given that any population, no matter how small, is a part of a larger population, some valid generalizations concerning the larger population may be formulated. That is to say, the nurses in one hospital are a part of a larger health care system which includes the community, the state, and the nation. "As each level is explored, greater strength and depth will be added to the explanation of the social phenomenon under consideration" [7].

Qualitative Research Strategies

Qualitative researchers employ a variety of strategies to generate useful data related to the phenomena they are investigating. These methods include *phenomenology, ethnography,* and *grounded theory.*

Phenomenology

Phenomenologic research is based on the philosophy of phenomenology, which proposes to understand the response of the whole human being to a situation or situations. When this philosophy is translated into a research setting, several processes must occur:

1. A person must communicate an experience or series of experiences to the researcher.
2. The researcher attempts to translate the communicated experience into an understanding of the person's experience.
3. The researcher then breaks this understanding into the underlying concepts that are the themes of the experience.
4. The researcher communicates his or her understandings to an audience in writing so that the members of this audience can then relate their understanding of this information to past and future experiences.

Because of the potentially large amount of data to be gathered and analyzed, phenomenologic research is usually based on data gathered from a very small number of individuals. Note that phenomenologic research is based on the intuitive analysis of other persons' experiences and that this necessitates special training before the researcher can make valid analyses.

Ethnography

Ethnographic research, often described as "participant observation," has long been the domain of the cultural anthropologist. Such research requires that the researcher be physically present among the subjects during the data-gathering phase of the research process. The ethnographer attempts to describe the culture of a group through in-depth study, involving systematic observation of the group's activities, language, and customs.

Systematic observation requires that the researcher be in the field long enough to see deeply into the group being studied. The procedures for observing and recording data are reported so that other field workers can attempt to replicate the study. Systematic observation is methodical; that is, strategies for observation are carefully laid out prior to the study. Even with such strategies in place, the researcher must be flexible enough to change methods of observation (and document such change) if the study setting requires it.

Ethnographic research has been further divided into a series of subresearch strategies, which have been called *ethnomethodology.* Ethnomethodology is similar to phenomenology in that it involves an attempt to understand how people see, describe, and explain the world in which they live. Ethnomethodologists base their explanatory systems on analysis of the speech and the activities of groups rather than attempting to understand the perceptions of individuals, as is done in phenomenology. This kind of data analysis leads to explanations of the commonsense understandings that groups of individuals hold.

Grounded Theory

Grounded theory is a research strategy that generates the theoretical underpinnings of the research being done by "grounding" or basing the theory on the data being collected. The grounded theorist determines the research question by observing how people solve problems in a social setting.

Grounded theory can be used in situations or areas where there has been little previous research, making it extremely difficult to test a previously developed theoretical position. Consequently, the grounded theorist uses the *inductive method* of developing theory while in the process of collecting data. This is in contrast to the *deductive method* of developing theory, in which theory is used to guide data collection and analysis.

As the researcher collects data, using a variety of data collection techniques such as observation, interviews, and questionnaires, each datum (a unit of data) is reviewed and compared to all of the other data. By using this comparative strategy, the researcher begins intuitively to develop concepts concerning the data. That is, the data are placed in categories; certain data fit into one category and other data fit into other categories.

After the data are categorized and concepts emerge, the researcher begins to analyze the data deductively. Theories are developed, and hypotheses based on these theories can be tested either quantitatively or qualitatively. As hypotheses are rejected, the concept that is the most important to theory development emerges. Finally, the data are again compared to the emergent theory so that the theory can be tested and modified to conform with known data.

Summary

In this chapter, we have considered selected aspects of the quantitative and qualitative traditions of scientific inquiry. Both have provided—and will continue to provide—valuable strategies for investigating nursing problems. Neither approach is better than the other. The important point is that the researcher should use the approach that is the most appropriate for the particular purpose of the investigation.

References

1. Leininger, M. L., Ed. 1985. *Qualitative Research Methods in Nursing.* Orlando, FL: Grune and Stratton.
2. Omery, A. 1983. "Phenomenology: A Method for Nursing Research." *Advances in Nursing Science,* January, p. 62.

3. Ibid., p. 49.
4. Callow, L. B., and B. Pieper. 1989. "Effect of Backrest on Central Venous Pressure in Pediatric Cardiac Surgery." *Nursing Research,* 38 (November–December): 336–338.
5. Leininger, *Qualitative Research Methods,* p. 14.
6. Field, P. A., and J. Morse. 1985. *Nursing Research: The Application of Qualitative Approaches.* Rockville, MD: Aspen, p. 122.
7. Dobbert, M. L. 1982. *Ethnographic Research.* New York: Praeger, p. 180.

Bibliography and Suggested Readings

Aamodt, A. 1982. "Examining Ethnography for Nurse Researchers." *Western Journal of Nursing Research,* 4 (Spring): 209–221.

Berry, J. W. 1980. "Introduction to Methodology." In H. C. Triandis and J. W. Berry, Eds., *Handbook of Cross-Cultural Psychology, Volume 2: Methodology.* Boston: Allyn and Bacon, pp. 1–28.

Bowens, E. 1994. "Ethnomethodology: An Approach to Nursing Research." *International Journal of Nursing Studies,* 29: 59–67.

Callow, L. B., and B. Pieper. 1989. "Effect of Backrest on Central Venous Pressure in Pediatric Cardiac Surgery." *Nursing Research,* 38 (November–December): 336–338.

Dobbert, M. L. 1982. *Ethnographic Research.* New York: Praeger.

Field, P. A., and J. M. Morse. 1985. *Nursing Research: The Application of Qualitative Approaches.* Rockville, MD: Aspen.

Fielding, N. G., and R. M. Lee, Eds. 1991. *Using Computers in Qualitative Research.* Newbury Park, CA: Sage.

Leininger, M., Ed. 1985. *Qualitative Research Methods in Nursing.* Orlando, FL: Grune and Stratton.

Lincoln, Y. S., and E. G. Guba. 1985. *Naturalistic Inquiry.* Beverly Hills, CA: Sage.

Lindzey, G., and E. Aronson, Eds. 1985. *Handbook of Social Psychology,* 3rd ed. New York: Random House.

Morse, J. M., Ed. 1989. *Qualitative Nursing Research: A Contemporary Dialogue.* Rockville, MD: Aspen.

Munhall, P. L., and C. O. Boyd. 1993. *Nursing Research: A Qualitative Perspective,* 2nd ed. New York: National League for Nursing Press.

Omery, A. 1983. "Phenomenology: A Method for Nursing Research." *Advances in Nursing Science,* January: 49–63.

Pelto, J. P., and G. Pelto. 1978. *Anthropological Research,* 2nd ed. Cambridge: Cambridge University Press.

Polkinghorne, D. 1983. *Methodology for the Human Sciences: Systems of Inquiry.* Albany, NY: State University of New York Press.

Porter, E. J. 1989. "The Qualitative-Quantitative Dualism." *Image,* 21 (Summer): 98–102.

Sarter, B., Ed. 1988. *Paths to Knowledge: Innovative Research Methods for Nursing.* New York: National League for Nursing.

Streubert, H. J., and D. R. Carpenter. 1995. *Qualitative Research in Nursing: Advancing the Humanistic Imperative.* Philadelphia: J. B. Lippincott Company.

Triandis, H. C., and J. W. Berry, Eds. 1980. *Handbook of Cross-Cultural Psychology, Volume 2: Methodology.* Boston: Allyn and Bacon.

Tripp-Reimer, T., and M. C. Dougherty. 1985. "Cross Cultural Nursing Research." In H. H. Werley and J. J. Fitzpatrick, Eds., *Annual Review of Nursing Research.* New York: Springer.

Werner, O., and G. M. Schoepfle, Eds. 1987. *Systematic Fieldwork.* Beverly Hills, CA: Sage.

Werley, H. H., and J. J. Fitzpatrick, Eds. 1985. *Annual Review of Nursing Research.* New York: Springer.

4   Ethical Considerations for Protection of Human Subjects in Research

Objectives

When you have finished reading this chapter you should be able to:

1. Discuss the development of ethical codes

2. Discuss the purpose of institutional review boards

3. Identify the components of appropriate informed consent

4. Discuss why some kinds of research cannot have prior informed consent

---

> **Development of Ethical Codes**
> **Institutional Review Boards**
> **Informed Consent**

In Chapter 1 we discussed the basic tenets of the scientific method and presented a brief history of nursing research. Chapter 2 provided an overview of the research process. In Chapter 3, quantitative and qualitative methodologies were compared and discussed. The purpose of this chapter is to acquaint you with one of the most important considerations of research that involves human subjects. This is the field of ethics in research.

Development of Ethical Codes

Researchers working with humans must always remember that their subjects are real people with their own needs and wants, not just numbers on a piece of paper. To this end, codes of ethics for human subject research have been developed to ensure the protection of the subjects' dignity and safety and the worthiness of research involving human subjects. These ethical codes are based on the Articles of the Nuremberg Tribunal, which were drawn up after the trials of the Nazi doctors accused of war crimes during the "doctor trials" following World War II. The defense that these individuals brought forward was that they were engaged in important research regardless of the pain and suffering they caused in their helpless subjects. The articles serve as a standard against which to measure the individual rights of subjects participating in experimental and clinical research.

The Nuremberg Code includes the following points:

1. The voluntary consent of the human subject is absolutely essential.
2. The experiment should be such as to yield fruitful results . . . and not random or unnecessary. . . .
3. The experiment should be based on . . . [prior knowledge] and the anticipated results should justify . . . the experiment.
4. The experiment should . . . avoid all unnecessary physical and mental suffering and injury.
5. No experiment should be conducted where there is an a priori reason to believe that death or disabling injury will occur; except . . . where the experimental physicians also serve as subjects.
6. The degree of risk should never exceed . . . the importance of the problem to be solved. . . .
7. Proper preparations should be made and adequate facilities provided to protect . . . subject(s) against . . . possibilities of injury, disability, or death.
8. The experiment should be conducted only by scientifically qualified persons.
9. During the course of the experiment, the human subject should be able to bring the experiment to an end. . . .
10. During the course of the experiment the scientist must be prepared to terminate the experiment if he has probable cause . . . that a continuation of the experiment is likely to result in injury, disability or death to the experimental subject. [1]

In 1964 the World Medical Assembly adopted a code of ethics that has become known as the Declaration of Helsinki. This code was based on the Nuremberg Code and was revised to provide further protection of human subjects in 1975.

The U.S. Department of Health and Human Services has provided a set of guidelines that researchers who are funded by the department must follow when using human subjects [2]. These guidelines require that an institutional review board (IRB) be established to ensure that the following conditions are met:

1. Risks to subjects are minimized by sound research procedures that do not expose subjects to risk unnecessarily. That is, projects using human

subjects should be so well thought out that the potential for unforeseen harm, either physical or psychological, should be minimized.

2. The anticipated benefits to subjects should outweigh the risks to the subjects, and knowledge to be gained should be of sufficient importance to merit any risks to which subjects might be subjected.

3. The rights and welfare of the subjects are adequately protected. That is, the researcher must terminate the research if subjects are being deprived of a procedure that might benefit them or are being subjected to one that is causing more harm than was anticipated.

An example of researchers terminating an experimental study in order to allow all subjects in the study to benefit would be the case in which it was determined that significantly lower doses of an expensive drug were just as effective and caused fewer side effects in patients who tested positive for a disease but who had not shown any symptoms. An example of researchers terminating a project because of unanticipated negative consequences would be the case of a social-psychological experiment in which subjects were placed in an uncomfortable situation and the experimenters noticed increasingly negative behaviors in the subjects that could be directly attributed to the experimental treatment.

4. The activity will be periodically reviewed by the institutional review board.

5. Informed consent has been obtained and appropriately documented. This is such an important area of concern that it will be discussed in greater detail in a later section of this chapter.

The 1985 *Human Rights Guidelines for Nurses in Clinical and Other Research,* published by the American Nurses' Association, outlines the responsibilities of nurses in practice, education, and research for safeguarding the rights of human subjects in research [3]. This document details three basic rights:

1. *The right to freedom from intrinsic risk of injury:* As mentioned in the previous discussion, subjects must be protected from physical, social, or emotional injury.

2. *The right to privacy and dignity:* Researchers should make every attempt to avoid invading their subjects' privacy and/or placing them in demeaning or dehumanizing situations.

The right to privacy also carries over to a patient's records. The Privacy Act of 1974 specifically denies the opening of records to unauthorized individuals. At times, however, a bona fide researcher needs to have access to existing records. Some states have established laws to protect the privacy of individuals, which include access to medical records; other states have not developed such statutes.

Many agencies have developed a prior consent or release of information form, which the potential subject signs as a routine part of obtaining whatever care is being provided. Without such prior consent, however, in many cases, the institutional review board may grant access to records when the board is certain that patient confidentiality will be respected and that only authorized investigators will have access to the records.

3. *The right to anonymity:* The identity of subjects participating in a study must not be disclosed, nor should the identity of individuals be recognizable through discussion or publication of the researchers' results, including photographs of the subject(s). If a subject's identity can be determined from the research, the researcher must have consent from the subject in order to include the information gained from that subject's participation.

The subjects of research include patients and outpatients, persons who are donors of organs and tissues, research volunteers, and volunteers with limited freedom—members of groups vulnerable to exploitation. This last category includes prisoners, residents of institutions for the mentally ill and mentally retarded, military personnel, and students [4].

Institutional Review Boards

As a result of the increasing awareness of ethical decision making in human research over the years, as well as the need to conform to the federal guidelines previously cited, most institutions sponsoring human subject research have a review group or committee whose responsibility is to ensure that researchers do not engage in unethical behavior or conduct poorly designed research. Membership on an IRB should include professionals who represent the discipline(s) from which the research framework is drawn, as well as representatives from the community at large. This means that the IRB in a hospital should include nurses as well as other health professionals and that the nursing representatives should have an equal voice in the deliberations of the committee.

Informed Consent

The greatest concern in human subject research is the protection of the subject's right of self-determination by the assurance of informed consent. This means that the subject must be made fully aware of the study and agree to participate in it. The need for this type of agreement may seem self-evident, but a large number of studies have been carried out without the participants' consent. A glaring and tragic example of such research in the United States is the study of black males with syphilis initiated in 1932 by the U.S. Public Health Service. This research project was designed to study the long-term effects of untreated syphilis in a sample of semiliterate black men in Macon County, Alabama. Specific treatment for the disease was withheld from a sample of 399 black males who had been diagnosed as having syphilis. The research subjects thought they were receiving treatment for "bad blood," which the researchers mistakenly thought was a term recognized by the subjects as meaning syphilis. Their progress was compared to that of a control group of 201 black males who did not have the disease. The so-called researchers then intended to follow the subjects through the rest of their lives to determine the long-term effects of untreated syphilis so that the "natural course" of the disease could be observed. Even though mortality rates were twice as high for the subjects with syphilis by the mid-1940s and continued to be higher than mortality rates for the control group, the U.S. Public Health Service did not provide treatment for the infected subjects until the research was exposed in 1972—40 years after the experiment began [5]. In 1980, when the first edition of this book was written, the survivors were still being sought, and large amounts of monetary compensation were being given to them and their survivors. In this case, there was no excuse for not obtaining informed consent from the subjects of the study; the cost in suffering and disability can never be justified.

Another example of failure to either obtain informed consent or of obtaining inadequate informed consent from human subjects can be shown in experiments using radioactive materials conducted by various U.S. government agencies during the 1940s, 1950s, and 1960s. There have been numerous investigations of these experiments. Some of the agencies that did obtain informed consent have been cited for providing inadequate information about the nature of their experiments and for failing to protect their subjects from harm. Clearly, this basic requirement of informed consent demonstrates that an investigator must not only plan for the present but must also consider the possibility of future re-examination when conducting experiments.

Essentially, the informed consent of subjects consists of the following six elements: (1) An explanation of the purpose of the study; (2) An explanation of potential risks and discomforts; (3) An explanation of potential benefits; (4) An acknowledgment that researchers will answer any questions the subjects may have concerning the study; (5) An acknowledgment that subjects can withdraw at any time; and (6) An assurance of anonymity and confidentiality.

1. *Subjects must be given an understandable explanation of the purpose of the study.* Subjects should also be told of the procedures and techniques that will be followed. In addition, experimental procedures and techniques should be identified. It may, however, be difficult to fulfill this requirement. As we point out in Chapter 9, subjects' awareness of the nature of the research or experiment may affect the experiment. There are those who suggest that a researcher cannot get a true random sample of a population, because once the subjects consent to be part of an experiment, it automatically means that the subjects in the experimental study are different from those individuals who refused to participate.

2. *Each subject should be given an explanation of the potential risks and discomforts he or she may encounter as a result of the study.* Will the subject be exposed to a potentially harmful situation? Withholding medication or treatment may cause physical or psychological distress to the subject. Further, withholding treatment may actually expose the subject to physical risks. Each subject must know the hazards he or she may face, if part of the study. Additionally, the right of personal privacy and dignity for each subject must be assured.

3. *Subjects should be told what benefits to expect.* The benefits can be a broad explanation; they may be the basis for an appeal to the subject's altruism, or merely a simple explanation. The intent of many experiments is to improve the human condition. Each time a new treatment is tried, it is usually believed to be more effective than existing modalities. Subjects must also be told of alternative procedures that would be advantageous to them. For example, in the case of the use of an experimental drug, subjects must be aware that other, already proven drugs may aid in their treatment, while the experimental drug may do nothing at all. Subjects must also be informed if benefits are to be withheld from them.

4. *Researchers must be willing to answer any questions the subjects may have about the procedures.* Most subjects want to know what is happening and why it is happening. In a research situation, subjects must be informed of what is happening, if they request such information.

5. *Subjects must be made aware that they can withdraw from the research investigation at any time without prejudice to their care.* Researchers cannot compel or coerce subjects to remain in any investigation against their will.

6. *Anonymity and confidentiality must be assured.* Subjects must be assured that any results will not be linked to them and that their responses will be kept confidential.

Unfortunately, the doctrine of informed consent cannot be followed to its fullest in many kinds of research. In the case of qualitative research, much of the research is done in such a way that there is no simple way to explain the nature of the research project, or the explanations may become so broad as to be meaningless. A researcher who simply states to the research subjects that he or she would find it interesting to see how people live their daily lives is not giving those subjects a great deal of information.

Also, it is not uncommon for researchers to be deceptive in their research strategy. This is especially true in psychological studies, where informing subjects of the true nature of the study could bias the results of the study. A classic example of such deception was a study conducted by Milgram [6]. In this study, subjects were told that they were involved in an experiment that proposed to measure the impact of punishment on a person's ability to learn. The subjects were to read a list of words to another person who, unbeknownst to the subjects, was the experimenter's confederate. If the confederate gave a wrong response, the subject was to "punish" the mistake by delivering an increasingly higher level of electric shock. The subject believed, incorrectly, that the confederate could receive a shock as high as 450 volts. Each subject was assured that no "permanent" damage would be done to the "learner." The confederate, however, who did not receive any shock at any time, feigned great pain as the administered shocks increased in strength. When the subject protested about administering pain, he was told to continue by the experimenter—the voice of authority. A very high degree of obedience to authority was obtained, and the study demonstrated how ordinary individuals might engage in harmful activities if urged to do so by those perceived to have authority over them. It is important to note that each subject was debriefed after the experiment was conducted and was shown that the confederate—the "victim"—was not actually harmed and had, in fact, received no shocks.

When this study was first published, it created an ethical controversy concerning the use of deception with study subjects, and the Milgram study still remains controversial. As a consequence of this and other studies requiring deception, many institutional review boards now demand that if the research design involves any form of deception, the researcher must provide a strong rationale for such deception and present a plan that allows for adequate debriefing of the study's subjects after the experiment's conclusion.

Another example of deception in research that has generated a great deal of ethical controversy is contained in the work of Humphreys [7]. In this study, published in 1970, Humphreys observed a number of homosexual acts in public restrooms, known as "tearooms" to the participants. He assumed the role of "watchqueen" or lookout, with the responsibility for warning of danger while others performed homosexual acts. Later, by using names and addresses obtained from records of license plate numbers, Humphreys, who altered his appearance and claimed to be a health inspector, interviewed a number of his subjects in their homes. The results of the study showed that only a few of the individuals interviewed were members of the recognized homosexual community; many were married and did not consider themselves either homosexual or bisexual. They did, however, consider their marriages to be marked by tension.

Although Humphreys received the C. Wright Mills Award for outstanding research on a critical social issue, his work generated bitter controversy at the institution that awarded his Ph.D. degree. In fact, some members of the faculty attempted to void his degree because of the controversial nature of his research. Humphreys' work also created a stir in various newspaper columns throughout the country—an almost unheard-of event in the annals of academe.

The controversy generated by this study still lingers. A key issue is the right to privacy demanded when conducting a research study. Did Humphreys adhere to this concept when he obtained the names and addresses of the individuals involved from the license plates of their automobiles parked outside the "tearooms," or did he increase the possibility that they would be arrested? Another important consideration was his active participation as lookout in an illegal activity. Can the study of illegal behaviors be conducted as a value-free enterprise, and does the researcher thereby lend credibility to the activities?

In all research studies it is essential that the researcher be able to document that he or she has obtained the informed consent of the subject(s). Such consent is best obtained on a written form stating that the subject has willingly entered into the research project and is aware of the risks, procedures, and benefits involved. The following form might be used:

I _____ [subject] do agree to participate in a research/experimental study concerning _____. This project may expose me to _____ risks and attendant discomforts. I am aware that _____ might be advantageous to me in the treatment of my condition instead of the experimental treatment.

I may ask any questions about the procedures and treatments taking place and my questions must be answered honestly and fully.

I am free to withdraw this consent and discontinue participation in this research study at any time without this decision affecting me in any way.

I understand that my responses will be kept confidential and not linked to me in any way.

Name and phone number of investigator	Signature of subject Date

Oral consent is also valid but should be witnessed by a third party for the protection of both the researcher and the subject. In the event that the potential subjects are not able to give informed consent because of mental or physical disabilities, or because they are below the legal age of consent, the researcher must gain the consent of a legally authorized guardian or next of kin.

Upon completion of a research investigation involving human subjects, the researcher has the obligation to remove any harmful aftereffects, debrief the subjects if necessary, and follow through on any commitments made to the subject. This also includes the provision of any study results that have been promised.

Nurses have a professional obligation to become knowledgeable participants in health care practice and research, and to be sure that they involve themselves in institutional policymaking and review activities:

> Knowledge about the changing scope of nursing responsibility and the emerging ethical issues affecting all practitioners in health care today is necessary for a professional nursing practice that accepts accountability for the protection of the human rights of consumers. [8]

References

1. *Trials of War Criminals Before the Nuremberg Military Tribunals, Volumes I and II: The Medical Case.* 1948. As cited in J. Katz. 1972. *Experimentation with Human Beings.* New York: Russell Sage Foundation, pp. 305–306.
2. U.S. Department of Health and Human Services. 1981. "Basic HHS Policy for the Protection of Human Research Subjects." *Federal Register,* 46: 8366–8392.
3. American Nurses' Association. 1985. *Human Rights Guidelines for Nurses in Clinical and Other Research.* Code No. D-46 5M 2/85. Kansas City: American Nurses' Association, pp. 6–7.
4. Ibid., p. 7.
5. Jones, J. H. 1981. *Bad Blood.* New York: Free Press.
6. Milgram, S. 1974. *Obedience to Authority.* New York: Harper & Row.
7. Humphreys, L. 1970. *The Tearoom Trade.* Chicago: Aldine.
8. American Nurses' Association. *Human Rights Guidelines,* p. 16.

Bibliography and Suggested Readings

American Nurses' Association. 1985. *Human Rights Guidelines for Nurses in Clinical and Other Research,* Code No. D-46 5M 2/85. Kansas City: American Nurses' Association.

Anderson, G., and V. Anderson. 1987. *Health Care Ethics.* Germantown, MD: Aspen.

Applebaum, P. S., L. H. Roth, and T. Detre. 1984. "Researchers' Access to Patient Records: An Analysis of the Ethical Problems." *Clinical Research,* 32 (October): 399–403.

Cassell, J. 1980. "Ethical Principles for Conducting Fieldwork." *American Anthropologist,* 82: 28–41.

Department of Health and Human Services. 1981. "Basic HHS Policy for the Protection of Human Research Subjects." *Federal Register,* pp. 8366–8392.

Gortner, S. R. 1985. "Ethical Inquiry." In H. H. Werley and J. J. Fitzpatrick, Eds., *Annual Review of Nursing Research.* New York: Springer.

Humphreys, L. 1970. *The Tearoom Trade.* Chicago: Aldine.

Jones, J. H. 1981. *Bad Blood.* New York: Free Press.

Katz, J. 1972. *Experimentation with Human Beings.* New York: Russell Sage Foundation.

Levine, R. J. 1986. *Ethics and the Regulation of Clinical Research,* 2nd ed. Baltimore: Urban & Schwarzenberg.

Milgram, S. 1974. *Obedience to Authority.* New York: Harper & Row.

Murray, J. C., and R. A. Pagon. 1984. "Informed Consent to Research Publication of Patient-Related Data." *Clinical Research,* 32 (October): 404–408.

Ramos, M. C. 1989. "Some Ethical Implications of Qualitative Research." *Research in Nursing and Health,* 12 (February): 57–63.

Trials of War Criminals Before the Nuremberg Military Tribunals, Volume I and II: The Medical Case. 1948. Washington, DC: U.S. Government Printing Office.

Werley, H. H., and J. J. Fitzpatrick, Eds. 1985. *Annual Review of Nursing Research.* New York: Springer.

World Medical Assembly. 1975. *World Medical Association Declaration of Helsinki: Recommendations Guiding Medical Doctors in Biomedical Research Involving Human Subjects.* In R. J. Levine. 1986. *Ethics and the Regulation of Clinical Research,* 2nd ed. Baltimore: Urban & Schwarzenberg, pp. 427–429.

Part

II Applying the Scientific Process of Inquiry to Nursing Problems

The material in Part II is designed to acquaint you with the application of the scientific process of inquiry to nursing problems and presents principles and activities for applying the research process to nursing problems using both quantitative and qualitative methodologies.

Chapter 5 focuses on the selection and statement of the research problem, including a review of related literature, the formulation of a conceptual or theoretical framework, and a statement of the purpose of the study. Chapter 6 deals with data collection principles and techniques. Chapter 7 discusses historical data collection. Chapter 8 reviews methods of collecting data for descriptive research. Chapter 9 focuses on experimental methods in research. Chapter 10 discusses data analysis, and Chapter 11 focuses on the communication of research results.

5 Problem Selection and Statement

Objectives

When you have finished reading this chapter you should be able to:

1. Understand the process for selecting a researchable problem

2. Identify major sources of researchable problems

3. Specify criteria to evaluate a researchable problem

4. Discuss the purposes of a literature review

5. Understand the meaning and use of theoretical and conceptual frameworks

6. Identify the function of the statement of the purpose of the study

7. Specify three formats for stating the purpose of the study

8. Understand the meaning and functions of hypotheses

9. Describe the purpose for defining the terms used in the study

10. Understand the process for gaining competence in critiquing research using the process in this book

---

Selection of a Researchable Problem
Sources of Research Problems
Problem Selection Criteria
    Is the Topic Interesting?
    Is the Problem Researchable?
    Is the Problem Practicable?
    Is the Problem Significant?
    Is the Research Ethical?
Review of Related Literature
    Reasons to Review the Literature
Placing the Problem within a Theoretical or Conceptual
    Framework
    Theoretical Framework
    Conceptual Framework

In Chapter 2, the research process was described as a chain of reasoning that begins with a statement of the problem and systematically proceeds through the communication of the study's results.

The material in this chapter is designed to acquaint you with the initial step of the research process: selection and statement of the research problem. This is an extremely important component of the research process. It begins with the identification of a general problem area of interest and involves the subsequent narrowing down of the topic to a very specific problem to be investigated.

Selection of a Researchable Problem

The selection of the problem to be investigated is an extremely important step and determines to a large extent the nature and quality of the research. If you were to be asked to identify a research problem, it is helpful to think of the problem as a question needing to be answered or as a situation needing a solution. First, look at your professional experiences. Describe a situation that aroused your interest—even one that annoyed you—and led you to think that something ought to be done about it. Examples of general problem areas in nursing might include preoperative teaching for mastectomy patients, discharge planning for premature infants, successful breast feeding in primiparas, or medication errors made by posthospitalized geriatric patients. If you find that your own experience fails to generate a problem area, you could use the library for locating literature related to your area of professional interest.

Once you have identified a general problem area related to your interests and experience, you should narrow it down to one specific problem that is manageable within the research process. A problem that is too broad can result in a study that is too general or too difficult to conduct; the results may be hard to interpret. It is often helpful to state the problem as a question. For example, the general problem area of successful breast feeding in primiparas could be narrowed down by asking, "What is the effect of teaching about breast feeding to primiparas?" This might then generate more specific problems: "Are there differences in comparable success with breast feeding in primiparas taught specific concepts and techniques related to breast feeding versus primiparas not exposed to such teaching?" or "What is the effect of individualized versus group instruction on successful breast-feeding practices in primiparas?"

It is well worth the time and effort it takes to select a problem specific enough to result in a manageable study. In your efforts to narrow down a general problem area, however, be careful not to end up with a question so trivial that it is not worth the time and effort involved in researching it.

Sources of Research Problems

There are several major sources of problems that need to be researched. An obvious source is the researcher's own background and personal experiences. As a nurse, you are in an excellent position to identify researchable problems unique to nursing. For example, the research problem identified by the student who wrote the research proposal in Appendix B was the result of her own clinical observation. The student noticed that nurses caring for pediatric patients were being careless in their compliance with universal precautions guidelines, especially by not wearing gloves for intravenous sticks. She also observed that the younger and sicker the child, the less likely the nurses were to adhere to universal precautions.

Another important source of researchable topics is the literature. Research studies reported in various nursing and related journals provide many kinds of problems observed by other researchers. Many studies raise additional questions or include recommendations for further study that can form the basis of new studies. A study that has already been conducted can be replicated in a different setting to see if its findings can be generalized. For example, King and Tarsitano [1] conducted an approximate replication of the Lindeman and Van Aernam study [2], which investigated the effectiveness of structured and unstructured preoperative teaching in improving the ability of surgical patients to deep-breathe and cough postoperatively.

Investigation of problems derived from theory, a third source, can provide a meaningful contribution to scientific knowledge. Theory is not merely a body of facts; it provides an explanation of facts that is then used to explain or predict certain phenomena. A good theory can guide research by pointing to areas that need to be investigated. Research can also contribute to the related theory by confirming or failing to confirm some aspect of the theory:

> The more research is directed by scientific theory, the more likely are its results to contribute directly to the development and further organization of a scientific body of knowledge in nursing. [3]

It is necessary to be aware of both the sources of research problems and the importance of designing nursing research studies that contribute to nursing's scientific knowledge base.

Problem Selection Criteria

A researcher should evaluate the proposed problem and decide if it should be pursued through the research process by asking the following questions:

1. Is the topic of interest?
2. Is it researchable?
3. Is it practicable?
4. Is it significant?
5. Is it ethical to conduct research on this problem?

Is the Topic Interesting?

Because the researcher must become deeply involved in planning and implementing the research study, the topic should be one that will sustain interest over a prolonged period of time.

Is the Problem Researchable?

A researchable problem is one that can be investigated through the collection and analysis of data that exist in the real world. The meanings of the concepts must be clear and must be presented through tangible, observable evidence—that is, evidence obtained through direct observation or through other activities that will provide similar evidence relating to the concept.

Is the Problem Practicable?

A research problem is practicable if it is possible to carry out the necessary related activities. Once the researcher finds a topic of interest within his or her area of expertise, the following questions need to be considered:

1. Are appropriate methodology and resources available in terms of suitable measuring instruments or equipment?
2. Are subjects available?
3. Will the researcher have cooperation from others?

The length of time needed to complete the study and the cost involved also need to be considered.

Is the Problem Significant?

Even though a topic may be interesting in itself, the researcher must consider if it is sufficiently significant to warrant a study. A good nursing research problem should have practical and/or theoretical significance. Its solution should contribute to the improvement of nursing care or to the advancement of nursing as a profession by providing scientific knowledge and theoretical formulations.

The 1985 Priorities for Nursing Research developed by the American Nurses' Association Cabinet on Nursing Research can function as a guideline for selecting research problems. These priorities are listed in Table 5-1.

Is the Research Ethical?

Finally, the researcher must evaluate the ethical implications of the problem in order to protect the rights of the subjects who would participate in the study. Obtaining informed consent from participants, protecting them from harm, and maintaining anonymity and confidentiality are major considerations, as we pointed out in Chapter 4.

In summary, the selection of the research problem—the initial step in the research process—is extremely important and determines the nature and quality of the research study.

Review of Related Literature

The initial review of the literature helps to identify and state a research problem. The second review, involving the systematic identification and analysis of information pertaining to the specific problem selected for study, should be done during the initial stages of the research process. Unfortunately, some researchers fail to appreciate the importance of conducting the literature review at this point in the process. In their enthusiasm to proceed with the rest of the study, researchers fail to put the problem in the perspective of what has already been done.

Table 5-1. ANA Priorities for Nursing Research (1985)

1. Promote health, well-being, and ability to care for oneself among all age, social, and cultural groups.
2. Minimize or prevent behaviorally and environmentally induced health problems that compromise the quality of life and reduce productivity.
3. Minimize the negative effects of new health technologies on the adaptive abilities of individuals and families experiencing acute or chronic health problems.
4. Ensure that the care needs of particularly vulnerable groups, such as the elderly, children with congenital health problems, individuals from diverse cultures, the mentally ill, and the poor, are met in effective and acceptable ways.
5. Classify nursing practice phenomena.
6. Ensure that principles of ethics guide nursing research.
7. Develop instruments to measure nursing outcomes.
8. Develop integrative methodologies for the holistic study of human beings as they relate to their families and life-styles.
9. Design and evaluate alternative models for delivering health care and for administering health care systems so that nurses will be able to balance high quality and cost-effectiveness in meeting the nursing needs of identified populations.
10. Evaluate the effectiveness of alternative approaches to nursing education for the kind of practice that requires broad knowledge and a wide repertoire of skills, and for the kind of practice that requires specialized knowledge and a focused set of skills.
11. Identify and analyze historical and contemporary factors that influence the shaping of nursing professionals' involvement in national health policy development. [4]

From the American Nurses' Association, *Directions for Nursing Research: Toward the Twenty-first Century.* Kansas City, MO: American Nurses' Association Cabinet on Nursing Research, 1985. Reprinted with permission.

Reasons to Review the Literature

There are four primary reasons for conducting a literature review. The first is to determine what has already been done that relates to the problem. This helps avoid the duplication of previous studies and helps to develop a framework for the problem that relates it to completed studies. Because one of the aims of research in nursing is to develop theories of nursing, the literature search may provide a theoretical framework within which to investigate the problem. For example, theory related to learning might form the theoretical framework within which the problem of group versus individual instruction for breast feeding could be investigated.

Second, the literature review provides ideas about the kinds of studies that need to be done. Previous investigators and writers often make suggestions regarding problems that need further investigation. Reviewing the literature may stimulate the researcher to develop new insights into reported research or devise new problems to be investigated.

Third, the literature review serves to point out research strategies, specific research procedures, and information regarding measuring instruments that have been found to be productive as well as nonproductive for the problem. Capitalizing on the successes as well as the errors of other researchers helps the researcher to profit from and build on the experiences of other researchers.

Finally, the literature review can help the researcher to interpret the results of the study after it has been conducted by guiding the discussion of the findings in terms of agreement or nonagreement with other studies. Results that contradict the findings of other studies can suggest further studies to resolve such contradictions.

Placing the Problem within a Theoretical or Conceptual Framework

Beginning researchers are usually unnecessarily frightened or confused by the terms *theoretical framework* or *conceptual framework*. Several basic definitions should help. A *concept* is a single idea (often one word) that represents several related component ideas. Examples of concepts are *grief, alienation,* and *happiness.* Concepts are the basic ingredients of a *theory,* which in turn consists of a set of statements called *propositions,* which link the concepts. These are stated in such a way as to form a logically interrelated deductive system. Such a system allows for the logical production of new statements from the original set of propositions. A theory can be used to explain and/or predict events (phenomena). Examples of theories include Rotter's social learning theory, Festinger's cognitive dissonance theory, Selye's adaptation theory, and systems theory.

Theoretical Framework

The term *theoretical framework* simply means the use of one theory or interrelated theories to support the rationale (reason) for conducting the study and provide a guide to analyzing the results. For example, Ketefian investigated moral reasoning and moral behavior among practicing nurses within the theoretical framework of moral development formulated by Kohlberg [5].

Conceptual Framework

The term *conceptual framework* means the use of one or more related concepts that underlie the study problem and support the rationale (reason) for conducting the study. When one concept is used, it is the discussion of the component ideas within it that forms the basis for the conceptual framework. The concepts should also be discussed in relationship to the variables being investigated in the study. (A *variable* is an observation or measurement that can assume a range of values along some dimension.)

At this time in its development, nursing does not have well-defined and tested theories of nursing but, rather, various conceptual frameworks, which are also referred to as conceptual schemes or models, depending on the level of their development toward nursing theory. Examples of these formulations are Sister Callista Roy's model of adaptation, Dorothea Orem's model of self-care, and Martha Roger's framework based on the principle of homeodynamics. The student who wrote the research proposal in Appendix B used Imogene King's interacting systems framework for her study.

If nursing research is to make an essential contribution to the scientific knowledge base, quantitative researchers should place each study within a theoretical or conceptual framework so that new findings can be placed in the broader areas of already existing knowledge:

> Any one research project provides only a small bit of information, but these bits of information can eventually be brought together to form larger generalizations and conclusions, provided they are all conducted within the same frame of reference and directed toward the same end. [6]

Statement of the Purpose of the Study

The purpose of the study is the single statement that identifies the focus of the research. The purpose should state what the researcher intends to do to answer the research question that generated the problem being studied. Brink and Wood suggest that the statement of the research study's purpose can be written in three ways: (1) as a declarative statement, (2) as a question, or (3) as a hypothesis. The form depends on the way the research question is asked and the extent of the researcher's knowledge about the problem. The statement of the purpose should include information about what the researcher intends to do to collect data (such as observe, describe, or measure some variable), information about the setting of the study (where the researcher plans to collect the data), and information about who the study subjects will be [7].

The Purpose as a Declarative Statement

In our previously formulated question designed to describe the relationship between the type of teaching and success in breast feeding by primiparas, the purpose of the study written as a declarative statement could read: "The purpose of this study is to describe the effect of structured individualized versus structured group instruction on successful breast feeding by primiparas in their home setting." Note that the statement includes information about what the researcher intends to do (to describe), the setting of the study (home setting), and the subjects of the study (primiparas).

The Purpose as a Question

The purpose of the study, written as a question, could read: "The purpose of this study is to answer the question: Is there a significant relationship between a method of teaching about breast feeding and successful breast feeding by primiparas in their home setting?" Methods of teaching might include structured individual teaching, structured group teaching, and unstructured (incidental) teaching. The primiparas in the study could be interviewed regarding their perceptions of their own success with breast feeding and their satisfaction with the method of teaching to prepare them for breast feeding.

The Purpose as a Hypothesis

The purpose of the study, written as a hypothesis, could read: "The purpose of the study is to test the following hypothesis: Primiparas who receive individualized instruction in breast feeding will have a significantly more successful breast-feeding experience in their home setting than primiparas who receive structured group instruction in breast feeding."

More about Hypotheses

A *hypothesis* is simply a statement of predicted relationships between the variables being studied. It is often referred to as the researcher's "educated or calculated guess" as to the study question's answer. It should be supported by existing theory and previous research findings. A study may have more than one hypothesis (which are then referred to as *hypotheses*). In the statement of a hypothesis, an antecedent condition—called the *independent variable*—is related to the occurrence of another condition or effect, called the *dependent variable*. This can be shown as follows:

Condition X is related to the occurrence of *Condition Y*

Independent variable (antecedent condition)—
Dependent variable (effect)
or
Method of instruction on breast feeding—
Degree of success on breast feeding

To test the hypothesis, the researcher purposely manipulates the independent variable and attempts to control all the other conditions. The effect on the dependent variable, which occurs presumably as a result of the manipulation of the independent variable, is then noted. Thus, the independent variable comes first in time and is manipulated by the researcher. The dependent variable is the phenomenon that occurs as the researcher alters the independent variable.

Functions of the Hypothesis

Prior to the systematic review of the literature relevant to the research problem, researchers often have a tentative hypothesis or hypotheses that express an expectation of the outcome of their study. At this point in the research process, it is necessary to refine and finalize this hypothesis, since the hypothesis serves to narrow down the field of the research study and forces the researcher to be precise in stating the specific situation being studied. In addition, the hypothesis guides the methodology for the remainder of the study—that is, the collection of relevant data and the plan for analysis of the data. The hypothesis also serves as a framework for stating conclusions of the study as a direct answer to the purpose of the study. A good hypothesis will not only be consistent with theory and previous research, it will also be a reasonable explanation or prediction of the situation being studied. Finally, the hypothesis will be testable; that is, the researcher will be able to collect data that can then be analyzed statistically to determine if the hypothesis can be supported. A hypothesis is not proved; it is either supported or not supported (rejected).

Is a Hypothesis Always Necessary?

A hypothesis can be formulated only if the researcher has enough information to predict the study's outcome and intends to test the significance of the prediction. Although a hypothesis may specify a cause-and-effect relationship, most hypotheses specify a relationship between two or more variables. These variables may exist together, or a change in one will be associated with a change in the other. A hypothesis must be theoretically or conceptually based and is necessary in an experimental study that is designed to predict the relationship between variables. It is optional in a descriptive study in which the investigator describes what is, or may use the data to raise questions and/or generate hypotheses for further studies. Many historical research studies have hypotheses to examine the occurrence of events and conditions.

Classification of Hypotheses

You will hear the terms research hypothesis and statistical hypothesis used as classifications. A *research hypothesis* states the expected relationship between the variables that the researcher expects as the study's outcome. It is stated in the declarative form. The *statistical hypothesis* is also referred to as the *null hypothesis* because it is stated in the null form—that is, a statement of no difference or no relationship between the variables. This statement may not reflect the outcome expected by the researcher and thus may confuse the beginning researcher. It is used as a part of the decision-making procedures, which are statistically based. The null hypothesis exists because present statistical procedures generally cannot test the research hypothesis directly. For example, in the following research hypothesis, the researcher predicts the outcome of the study: "Primiparas who receive individualized instruction on breast feeding will have a more successful breast-feeding experience in their home setting than primiparas who receive group instruction on breast feeding." The following statistical hypothesis, stated in the null (no difference) form, does not reflect the outcome that is really expected by the researcher: "There will be no significant difference in the breast-feeding experience in their home setting between primiparas who receive individualized instruction on breast feeding and primiparas who receive group instruction on breast feeding."

Many researchers prefer to state the hypothesis in the null form because it reflects a more objective and scientific statement of the relationship between the variables. Also, the statistical procedures they plan to use to test the hypotheses may require the null form in order to determine whether an observed relationship is probably a chance relationship (due to sampling error, for example) or is probably a true relationship. The null form of the hypothesis, however, often does not reflect the researcher's true prediction of the study's outcome. And statements in the null form make it difficult to tie the hypothesis back to the background and theory of the research. Other researchers, therefore, prefer to use the research hypothesis, in which case the underlying null hypothesis is usually assumed without being explicitly stated.

Stating the Hypothesis

Brink and Wood provide guidelines for writing a hypothesis [8]. The hypothesis to test the relationship between method of instruction about breast feeding and a successful breast-feeding experience was stated as: "Primiparas who received structured individualized instruction in breast feeding will have a significantly more successful breast-feeding experience in their home setting than primiparas who receive structured group instruction in breast feeding." The first clause of the hypothesis identifies both the sample (primiparas) and one position of the independent variable (method of instruction on breast feeding, specified here as "structured individualized instruction"). The next clause specifies the expected direction of the dependent variable (degree of success on breast feeding, specified here as "more successful"). The final clause of the hypothesis specifies the other portion of the independent variable (specified here as "structured group instruction in breast feeding").

Gay suggests a general paradigm or model for stating research hypotheses (predictions of differences between variables) for experimental studies [9].

X's who get Y do better on Z than X's who do not get Y (or get some other Y).
In this model X's are the subjects.
Y is the treatment (independent variable).
Z is the outcome (dependent variable).

For example, "Primiparas (X's, subjects) who receive individualized instruction on breast feeding (Y, the treatment) will have a more successful breast-feeding experience in their home setting (Z, observed outcome) than primiparas who receive group instruction (get some other Y, treatment)."

When this model is applied to the null hypothesis previously stated, it looks like this: "There will be no significant difference in the breast-feeding experience in their home setting (Z, expected outcome) between primiparas (X's, subjects) who receive individualized instruction on breast feeding (Y, the treatment) and primiparas who receive group instruction on breast feeding (some other Y, treatment)."

Another form for a research hypothesis is the "If . . . then" form: "*If* primiparas receive individualized instruction on breast feeding, *then* they will have a more successful breast-feeding experience in their home than primiparas who receive group instruction." Any of these formats should help you write a statement that is truly a hypothesis.

In summary, although a hypothesis may be stated in different ways, the hypothesis statement should be in the form of an answer to the question(s) proposed by the study. It should state an expected relationship, should be stated clearly and concisely, and should be based on an accepted theory and/or valid research findings when possible. It must also be testable; that is, the researcher formulates a hypothesis for a research study in order to accept or to reject it statistically. The researcher must be able to collect and analyze data in such a way as to determine the validity of the hypothesis. Remember, a hypothesis is either *supported* or *rejected,* it is never proved or not proved.

The success of a research study does not depend on the hypothesis being supported by the data. A well-designed and well-executed research study in which the hypothesis is not supported can add just as much to the knowledge base, and to the theory from which it was derived, as a well-designed and well-executed study where the hypothesis was supported.

Definition of Terms

Just as the conceptual or theoretical framework and the hypothesis stem from the literature review, so do the definitions of the terms used in the study. The words in the statement of the study's purpose pertaining to the variables of the study should be defined either directly, operationally, or theoretically. A direct definition is the definition found in a dictionary. The other two types of definitions are discussed in this section.

Operational Definitions

An *operational definition* provides a full description of the method by which the concept will be studied. This is stated in behavioral, observable, demonstrable terms by citing the *operations* (the manipulations and observations) necessary to produce the phenomenon. For example, in the previously described statement of the purpose of the study, "the purpose of this study is to describe the effect of structured individualized versus structured group instruction on successful breast feeding by primiparas in their home setting," the variables to be defined include structured individualized instruction, structured group instruction, successful breast feeding in a home setting, and primiparas. "Structured individualized instruction" might be defined as a one-to-one instructional relationship between the professional nurse and the primipara, where a planned teaching protocol is used consistently. "Structured group instruction" might be defined as instruction of several primiparas by the nurse, where a planned teaching protocol is used consistently. "Successful breast feeding in a home setting" might be defined as the duration of breast feeding (weeks or months) or as the degree to which difficulties with home breast feeding were identified as problematic on a questionnaire administered to the mother 6 weeks after delivery. These are all operational definitions. "Primipara" can be defined directly by the definition found in a dictionary.

Theoretical Definitions

A *theoretical definition* of a variable uses the definition found in the specific language of the theory or theories being used in the study. For example, in cognitive dissonance theory, anxiety is defined as "the component of dissonance related to a state of drive or need or tension" [10].

A Note on Critical Evaluation of Published Research

The Council of Nurse Researchers of the American Nurses' Association (1993) has recommended that education in research at the undergraduate level should prepare the nurse to read research critically and to use existing standards to determine the readiness of research for utilization in clinical practice [11]. This entails the reading, understanding, and interpretation of published research studies to determine the study's scientific merit and application to practice.

In order to give you a systematic experience in learning the skills to become a critical consumer, you will read three published research reports dealing with the same research topic. As you learn each step in the research process, the Workbook Activities will direct you to read and evaluate the corresponding section of each research report. Eventually, you will have read—and evaluated—all sections of the three reports. This process is designed to develop your skills as a competent consumer of published research as well as to prepare you for the process of research utilization presented in Chapter 12.

The Workbook Activities for this chapter will help you evaluate your understanding of the material related to the selection and statement of a research problem and will assist you in beginning to develop your skills in evaluating published research.

References

1. King, I., and B. Tarsitano. 1982. "The Effect of Structured and Unstructured Pre-Operative Teaching: A Replication." *Nursing Research,* 31 (November–December): 324–329.
2. Lindeman, C., and B. Van Aernam. 1971. "Nursing Intervention with the Presurgical Patient—The Effects of Structured and Unstructured Preoperative Teaching," *Nursing Research,* 20 (July–August 1971): 319–332.
3. Abdellah, F., and E. Levine. 1979. *Better Patient Care through Nursing Research,* 2nd ed. New York: Macmillan, p. 75.
4. American Nurses' Association Cabinet on Nursing Research. 1985. *Directions for Nursing Research: Toward the Twenty-first Century.* Kansas City: American Nurses' Association, pp. 2–3.
5. Ketefian, S. 1981. "Moral Reasoning and Moral Behavior among Selected Groups of Practicing Nurses," *Nursing Research,* 30 (May–June): 171–176.
6. Fox, D. J. 1982. *Fundamentals of Research in Nursing.* Norwalk, CT: Appleton-Century-Crofts, p. 32.
7. Brink, P. J., and M. J. Wood. 1994. *Basic Steps in Planning Nursing Research,* 4th ed. Boston: Jones and Bartlett, p. 68.
8. Ibid., p. 78.
9. Gay, L. R. 1987. *Educational Research: Competencies for Analysis and Application,* 3rd ed. Columbus, OH: Charles E. Merrill, p. 57.
10. Silva, M. C. 1981. "Selection of a Theoretical Framework." In S. Kram-

pitz and N. Pavlovich, Eds., *Readings for Nursing Research*. St. Louis: C. V. Mosby, p. 19.

11. American Nurses' Association Council of Nurse Researchers. 1993. *Position Statement on Education for Participation in Nursing Research*. Washington, DC: American Nurses' Association, p. 1.

Bibliography and Suggested Readings

Abdellah, F., and E. Eugene. 1979. *Better Patient Care through Nursing Research,* 2nd ed. New York: Macmillan.

American Nurses' Association. 1975. *Human Rights Guidelines for Nurses in Clinical and Other Research.* Code No. D-465M. Kansas City: American Nurses' Association.

———. 1981. *Guidelines for the Investigative Function of Nurses.* Code No. D-69 3M. Kansas City: American Nurses' Association.

———. Cabinet on Nursing Research. 1985. *Directions for Nursing Research: Toward the Twenty-first Century.* Kansas City: American Nurses' Association.

———. Council of Nurse Researchers. 1993. *Position Statement on Education for Participation in Nursing Research.* Washington, DC: American Nurses' Association.

Brink, P. J., and M. Wood. 1994. *Basic Steps in Planning Nursing Research,* 4th ed. Boston: Jones and Bartlett.

Dempsey, P. 1977. "Improving Basic Library Skills." *Nursing Research,* 26 (September–October): 390.

Dickson, G., and H. Lee-Villasenon. 1982. "Nursing Theory and Practice: A Self-Care Approach." *Advances in Nursing Science,* 5 (October): 29–40.

Fawcett, J. 1993. *Analysis and Evaluation of Nursing Theories.* Philadelphia: F. A. Davis.

Field, P. A., and J. M. Morse. 1985. *Nursing Research: The Application of Qualitative Approaches.* Rockville, MD: Aspen Systems.

Fitzpatrick, J., and A. Whall. 1989. *Conceptual Models of Nursing: Analysis and Application,* 2nd ed. Norwalk, CT: Appleton and Lange.

Fox, D. J. 1982. *Fundamentals of Research in Nursing,* 4th ed. New York: Appleton-Century-Crofts.

Gay, L. R. 1987. *Educational Research: Competencies for Analysis and Application,* 3rd ed. Columbus, OH: Charles E. Merrill.

Ketefian, S. 1981. "Moral Reasoning and Moral Behavior among Selected Groups of Practicing Nurses." *Nursing Research,* 30 (May–June): 171–176.

Kim, H. 1983. "Use of Rogers' Conceptual System in Research." *Nursing Research,* 32 (March–April): 89–91.

King, I., and B. Tarsitano. 1982. "The Effect of Structured and Unstructured Preoperative Teaching: A Replication." *Nursing Research,* 31 (November–December): 324–329.

Krampitz, S., and N. Pavlovich. 1981. *Readings for Nursing Research.* St. Louis: C. V. Mosby.

Lindeman, C., and B. Van Aernam. 1971. "Nursing Intervention with the Presurgical Patient—The Effects of Structured and Unstructured Preoperative Teaching." *Nursing Research,* 20 (July–August): 319–332.

Morgan, J., et al. 1985. "Effects of Preoperative Teaching on Postoperative Pain: A Replication and Expansion." *International Journal of Nursing Studies,* 22: 267–280.

Polit, D., and B. Hungler. 1995. *Nursing Research: Principles and Methods,* 5th ed. Philadelphia: J. B. Lippincott.

Silva, M. C. 1981. "Selection of a Theoretical Framework." In S. Krampitz and N. Pavlovich, Eds., *Readings for Nursing Research.* St. Louis: C. V. Mosby.

6 Data Collection

Objectives

When you have finished reading this chapter you should be able to:

1. Differentiate between quantitative and qualitative forms of data

2. Differentiate between the three commonly used research approaches

3. Discuss the factors to be considered in choosing the appropriate data collection technique(s) for a research study

4. List the three basic attributes of quantitative data collection research instruments

5. Define the terms reliability and validity and explain the difference between them

6. Discuss three major approaches for estimating the validity of a quantitative measuring instrument

7. Discuss the four main types of reliability of a measuring instrument that may be determined through correlation

8. Explain the differences in the validity and reliability of data collection instruments in quantitative and qualitative research studies

9. Define the term and discuss the purposes for sampling

10. Distinguish between the two main approaches to sampling in quantitative research studies

11. Discuss the major methods of probability and nonprobability sampling

12. Explain the major considerations in determining sample size in a quantitative study

13. Discuss three sampling techniques for a qualitative research investigation

14. Understand the importance of stating assumptions and limitations for a research study

The Nature of Data
The Research Approach
  Differences between Research Approaches
  Selecting the Research Approach
Data-Gathering Techniques
Characteristics of Quantitative Research Instruments
  Validity
  Reliability
  Usability
Considerations in Selecting a Measuring Instrument
Validity and Reliability in Qualitative Research
Selecting the Study Subjects for Quantitative Research
  The Target Population
  The Sample
  Purpose of Sampling
  Quantitative Sampling Approaches
  Probability Sampling Methods
  Nonprobability Sampling Methods
  Sample Size
Selecting the Study Subjects in Qualitative Research
Stating the Assumptions of the Study
Stating the Limitations of the Study

In the previous chapters, we have presented material on the application of the research process to nursing problems. In the problem selection and statement step of the research process, a researchable problem is selected for study. The material in this chapter acquaints you with the next step in the research process: development of the overall plan to collect the information directly related to the study problem.

The Nature of Data

Data are the raw materials from which all research reports are generated. The data collected may be gathered in quantitative (numerical) forms or in qualitative (verbal/descriptive) forms. In either case, the investigator's job is to be sure that the data gathered are accurate and amenable to appropriate analysis.

The Research Approach

In Chapter 1, we stated that the research approaches most commonly used can be classified as (1) descriptive (which includes surveys and qualitative strategies), (2) experimental (also termed explanatory), and (3) historical (also termed documentary).

Table 6-1. Differences between Research Approaches

Research Approach	Time Orientation	Control of Independent Variable by Investigator	Random Assignment to Treatment Condition
Historical	Past (examines "what was")	No	No
Descriptive	Present (describes "what is")	No	No
Experimental	Future (predicts "what will be")	Yes	Yes

Differences between Research Approaches

These approaches are differentiated by their time orientation and the extent to which the investigator has control over manipulating the independent variable. The *historical* approach is past-oriented in that it examines what has already occurred; the investigator has no control over manipulating the independent variable. The *descriptive* approach is present-oriented, describing what is. The investigator has no control over manipulating the independent variable. The *experimental* approach is future-oriented; it predicts what will occur. Here the investigator has control in manipulating the independent variable in the experimental setting, and subjects are randomly assigned (each individual is assigned a place in a group based on chance alone) to the treatment (experimental) condition specified in the study. The term *quasi-experimental* refers to a modification of the experimental approach in which the investigator may have control in manipulating the independent variable, although subjects are not randomly assigned to the treatment condition. Table 6-1 summarizes these differences between the approaches.

Selecting the Research Approach

You will also see the research approaches referred to as *research methods* or *research designs.* All these terms refer to the overall plan for eliciting information about the study problem. You remember that the research process has been described as a chain of reasoning beginning with the statement of the problem and proceeding systematically through the communication and utilization of the study results. From this it is evident that the statement of the problem section of the research plan guides the choice of the study's research approach. An important consideration in quantitative research is the extent to which the research problem fits the framework of existing knowledge and theory. Use of the experimental approach requires more extensive knowledge, a problem that is formulated within a theoretical base and the ability to predict the action of the variables.

The form in which the purpose of the study is stated also guides the choice of the research approach. In general, the declarative statement and question indicate a descriptive or historical approach, whereas the hypothesis indicates an experimental approach because the investigator has control in manipulating the independent variable. Although it is possible to have a hypothesis in the historical or descriptive approach, such a hypothesis is not tested by direct manipulation of the variables, as in the experimental setting, but by statistical manipulation of the existing data.

Thus, in the step-by-step chain of reasoning that characterizes the research process, the components of the statement of the problem and the form of the statement of the purpose guide the selection of the research approach.

Data-Gathering Techniques

We have seen that the research approach refers to the overall method for obtaining the study's data. Choice of the techniques for gathering the data depends on the nature and sources of the data to be collected. Many research studies use more than one technique for gathering data. For example, in a study designed to describe the learning achieved by student nurses when caring for terminally ill patients, learning could be measured in the cognitive, affective, and psychomotor domains. A paper-and-pencil test could be used to gather data measuring cognitive learning (knowledge); an interview schedule could be used to ascertain attitudes on the affective domain; and an observational checklist might be used to gather data on the student's technical proficiency in performing psychomotor skills (procedures).

The terms *continuous data* and *discrete data* are used to refer to quantitative variables. Continuous data can be located at some point along a continuum or scale and are characterized by fractional values of a whole unit. For example, 98.6°F, body temperature, is a point on the Fahrenheit scale used to measure body temperature. Discrete data, on the other hand, exist only in distinct units expressed as whole numbers that are precise and definite: 6 patients, 5 hospitals, 6 beds (not $6\frac{1}{2}$ patients, $5\frac{1}{4}$ hospitals, or $6\frac{2}{3}$ beds).

The decision as to which form to use to collect data depends on the nature of the study's research approach, the need for precision, and the availability of appropriate data collection instruments. One problem with quantification is the lack of instruments for collecting appropriate quantitative data. Nursing research is often concerned with such areas of study as wellness, illness, and reactions to various situations, which are not easily amenable to quantified measurements.

Characteristics of Quantitative Research Instruments

When we refer to research instruments or research tools, we are talking about devices or equipment used to gather the research data. Research instruments must possess certain basic attributes, which assure us that they will provide dependable measurements of the variables under investigation. The most important attributes are (1) validity, (2) reliability, and (3) usability.

Validity

Validity refers to the ability of a data-gathering instrument to measure what it is supposed to measure, to obtain data relevant to what is being measured. Validity is an extremely important characteristic of a measuring instrument. A clinical thermometer is a valid instrument for measuring an individual's body temperature, but a sphygmomanometer is not valid for this purpose. A yardstick is a valid instrument for measuring cloth, but a baby scale is not. In estimating the validity of a measuring instrument, the questions "Valid for what?" and "Valid for whom?" must be answered. In the case of measuring body temperature, the clinical thermometer is valid for measuring body temperature (what?) on human beings (whom?).

There are three main approaches for estimating the validity of a measuring instrument designed to collect quantitative data: content validity, construct validity, and criterion-related validity.

The *content validity* of a measuring instrument is the extent to which the instrument represents the factors under study. Each content area must be defined, and representative behaviors are then identified. A number of experts in the field of the specific study topic are then asked to examine each item and to make judgments regarding how well the items and the entire instrument reflect the previously defined content area(s). No statistical procedures are involved in determining the content validity of a measurement instrument. A subtype of content validity is *face validity,* which is determined by inspecting the items to see if the instrument contains important items that measure the variables in the content area. Face validity is the least time-consuming and least rigorous method for determining validity because it is based entirely on the subjective judgment of the investigator.

Construct validity is the degree to which a measuring instrument measures a specific hypothetical trait or *construct,* such as intelligence, grief, or prejudice. Establishing construct validity is a complicated and time-consuming process that requires the measuring instrument to be used in a succession of different studies that use various methods for testing construct validity. A basic approach to establishing construct validity is the *known-groups technique,* in which the instrument is administered to several groups known to differ on a certain construct. If the results obtained demonstrate statistically significant differences, as expected, then the instrument is said to have a degree of construct validity. For example, in establishing the construct validity of an instrument for measuring preoperative anxiety, it would be expected that the preoperative anxiety reported by a group of patients having minor surgery in an ambulatory care unit would differ from the preoperative anxiety reported by patients admitted to the hospital for major surgery. Other procedures for demonstrating construct validity (such as factor analysis) are discussed in more advanced research and statistics textbooks. Although construct validity is considerably more difficult to establish than content validity, it is important to establish construct validity when complex concepts are being measured.

Criterion-related validity refers to the relationship of the measuring instrument to some already known external criterion or other valid instrument. *Predictive validity* predicts how well a person will do in the future. For example, the scores received on the Graduate Record Examination (GRE) are supposed to predict a student's potential for success in graduate work in a college or university. *Concurrent validity* is a measure of how well an instrument correlates with another instrument that is known to be valid. For example, an individual's score on the Stanford-Binet IQ test should be very similar to that individual's score on the Wechsler intelligence test.

Reliability

The *reliability* of a measuring instrument refers to its ability to obtain consistent results when reused. An instrument is reliable when it consistently does whatever it is supposed to do in the same way. For example, when a paper-and-pencil test of intelligence is administered to an individual, the test should produce approximately the same result if it is readministered as a retest. The more reliable a measuring instrument is, the more confidence we can have that the scores obtained would not fluctuate too greatly from administration time to administration time.

Reliability is usually expressed as a number, called a *coefficient*. A high coefficient indicates a high reliability. A measuring instrument that has a perfect reliability would have a coefficient of 1.00. Rarely, however, is a measuring instrument perfectly reliable. Reliability is more often reported as less than 1.00—that is, .80, .70, or .50. Less than perfect reliability of an instrument can be due to errors in measurement, such as the conditions under which the instrument was administered (e.g., improper directions); problems with the instrument itself (e.g., poorly constructed items); or characteristics of the individuals responding to the instrument (e.g., illness or fatigue).

There are several main types of reliability that may be determined through *correlation:* (1) test–retest reliability, (2) alternate forms reliability, (3) split-half reliability, and (4) interrater reliability.

Test–retest reliability indicates variation in scores from one administration of the instrument to the next, resulting from measurement errors. The procedure for determining test–retest reliability is to administer the instrument to individuals similar to the ones you plan to study, let some period of time elapse (say a week) to allow for some loss of memory of the items, then give the instrument to the same individuals again. The scores on the two instruments are then correlated statistically to yield a coefficient referred to as the *coefficient of stability.* If the results are the same or similar, the coefficient will be high—say .90—and the instrument is said to have high test–retest reliability. One of the major problems with this method of estimating reliability is that of deciding realistically how long the time interval between the test and the retest should be. If the interval is too short, the individuals tend to remember their responses to the items on the first administration. This results in an artificially high coefficient of reliability. If the time interval is too long, some individuals may do better on a retest because of their own learning and maturation during the interval between the test and the retest.

Alternate forms reliability is also called "equivalent forms reliability." To establish this type of reliability, at least two different forms of the instrument are constructed. Although the actual items on the instruments are not the same, each form has the same number of total test items, is designed to measure the same variable or variables, and has the same level of difficulty. Both use the same procedures for administration, scoring, and interpreting results. At least two different forms of the instrument must be available. The procedure for determining alternate forms reliability is to administer one form of the test to a group of individuals and then, at the same session or very shortly thereafter, administer a second form to the same individuals. The two sets of scores are then statistically correlated, and the instrument has good alternate forms reliability if the correlation coefficient is high. There are two major problems with this method. One is the difficulty involved in constructing two forms that are equivalent; this can result in measurement errors. The second is the difficulty in administering two different instruments to the same individuals within a relatively short time period.

Split-half reliability, also called "odd–even reliability," yields the coefficient of internal consistency. This estimate of reliability requires only one administration of an instrument in order to estimate its reliability. The entire instrument is administered to a group of individuals, and then the responses for each individual are divided into two comparable halves: all the responses to even items in one half and all the responses to odd items in the other. The response score for each individual is then computed separately for the two halves, resulting in a response score for the even items and a response score for the odd items. The two sets of scores are then correlated statistically to yield a correlation coefficient. If this is high, the instrument is said to have good split-half reliability. This method is more effective for longer instruments. For an instrument consisting of a limited number of items, a correlation formula such as the Spearman-Brown prophecy formula must be applied. The split-half method of estimating reliability has the advantage of requiring only one administration and one form of the instrument; it also eliminates the problems associated with more than one administration of the instrument to the same individuals. Other common reliability coefficients are Cronbach's alpha and the Kuder-Richardson formula (K-R 20).

Interrater reliability is also called "interobserver reliability." Two or more different observers independently observe and record their observations using the same recording format. The strength of the agreement between the two sets of observations may be computed as a correlation.

Usability

The *usability* of a measuring instrument refers to the practical aspects of using it. These include ease of administration, scoring, and interpretation as well as financial, time, and energy considerations. It is important to an instrument's usability that these practical aspects be considered.

In summary, the three basic attributes of dependable quantitative research instruments or tools are (1) validity, (2) reliability, and (3) usability. Because the outcome of a research study depends on the instrument(s) used to collect the data, research instruments that meet these criteria increase the potential for high-quality research.

Considerations in Selecting a Measuring Instrument

Given that it takes a great deal of time and skill to develop a measuring instrument, researchers are well advised to select an appropriate instrument that has already been developed.

If using a self-developed instrument, the researcher can take parts from one or more instruments for use in developing the new instrument and must then pretest the new instrument on a group similar to the one to be used in the study. A *pretest* is the process of testing the effectiveness of the instrument in gathering the appropriate data by administering the instrument to subjects who meet the criteria for study subjects, and then evaluating the instrument's strengths and weaknesses and revising it as necessary.

Validity and Reliability in Qualitative Research

Qualitative researchers are also concerned with establishing validity and reliability during their data collection. However, the meanings of the terms differ for qualitative and quantitative research because the selection of the sample, the data collection, and the data analysis are carried out differently.

In qualitative research, *validity* refers to the extent to which the research findings represent reality [1]. The investigator must thoroughly check the information gathered to determine whether it makes sense when compared to other information that has been gathered. In a qualitative research study that uses multiple informants and accurate observation by the researcher, if all of the informants state that something is the case and the researcher observes that what the informants have stated either is not true or is somehow in conflict with observed behaviors, then the researcher must include this information in the research report and attempt to reconcile the differences. For example, if a researcher interviews nurses in a hospital setting and is told that they always perform certain activities, but then observes that these activities are either omitted or overelaborated, the researcher must attempt to determine why the differences between the reported and actual behavior occurred.

Reliability in qualitative research has two specific concerns. The first is that the information gathered from the research's informant(s) is accurate. This concern can cause problems because an informant either may not have sufficient information or may be lying. In order to reduce or eliminate these possibilities, the researcher must use a variety of informants, if possible, and must ask the questions crucial to the research in several different ways in order to determine whether the responses garnered are consistent.

Since the data-gathering instrument for a qualitative research study is often an interviewer or observer, the second concern related to reliability in qualitative research is the reliability of the data collector. If the data collector is careless or biased, the reliability of the study will be either substantially diminished or completely absent. One way to determine the reliability of a qualitative research study is to see if the research report gives enough documentation of the questions asked and the responses obtained so that another researcher could go to the same or a similar setting and obtain similar responses by asking the same questions.

Selecting the Study Subjects for Quantitative Research

An essential part of the data collection plan is the selection of the study subjects who will provide the necessary data in relation to the purpose of the study.

The Target Population

The investigator must delineate a *target population,* consisting of individual people or things that meet the designated set of criteria of interest to the researcher. In nursing research, the target population usually consists of humans. However, it can also consist of human characteristics (e.g., personality, job activities), inanimate objects (e.g., hospitals), or abstract concepts (e.g., professional ethics, community attitudes) [2].

The Sample

Because size, cost, time, or lack of accessibility often make it impossible to study the whole population directly, a study is usually done on a smaller part of a target population, called a *sample.* The term *sampling* refers to the process of selecting a number of individuals from the delineated target population in such a way that the individuals in the sample represent as nearly as possible the characteristics of the whole target population. The sample can be thought of as a miniature of the larger target population. A single unit or member of the target population is referred to as a *population element* or a *sampling unit.*

For example, a study proposes to investigate the effect of educational preparation on the political perceptions of all licensed nurses in the state of Florida. Because it would probably not be feasible to study such a large number of individuals, a sample of these nurses would be selected for inclusion in the study. This would be done in such a way that they would be representative of all the licensed nurses in Florida. Such a selection could be accomplished by first obtaining a computer listing of all the licensed nurses in the state from the Florida Board of Nursing. The investigator would then select a fraction of the licensed nurses on the list in such a way that those selected for inclusion in the study would be representative of all licensed nurses in Florida. Each licensed nurse in the sample would then be a population element and a sampling unit.

Purpose of Sampling

A basic purpose of sampling is to be able to use the sample's findings to generalize or extrapolate beyond the actual sampling units without having to study each element of the target population. The extent of this ability to generalize beyond the actual sampling units to the target population depends on the sampling approach used.

Quantitative Sampling Approaches

Sampling theory distinguishes between two main approaches to sampling in quantitative research: *probability sampling* and *nonprobability sampling.*

Probability Sampling

When using *probability sampling,* the investigator can specify, for each element of the population, the probability that it will be included in the sample. Usually each element has the *same* probability of being included in the sample, but the basic requirement is that there exists a *known* probability that a given element will be included. The sampling units are selected by chance, and neither the investigator nor the population elements have any conscious influence on what is included in the sampling.

Nonprobability Sampling

Nonprobability sampling does not enable the investigator to estimate the probability that each element of the population will be included in the sample or even that it has some chance of being included.

The importance of the ability to estimate probability lies in the interpretation of the study findings to the target population with a given degree of certainty. Probability sampling has the advantage of permitting the investigator to generalize from the sample's findings to the target population with a given degree of certainty. That is, these sample findings do not differ by more than a specific amount from the expected findings if the investigator were using the total population. Nonprobability samples do not permit generalization of the study findings from the sample to the population.

Choice of the sampling approach depends on the research problem and the purpose of the study. Not all studies are conducted with the purpose of being able to generalize to the entire population. The important point is that the sampling approach must be consistent with the purpose of the study.

Probability Sampling Methods

Major methods of probability sampling include (1) simple random sampling, (2) stratified random sampling, and (3) cluster sampling. The following discussion of each is intended to provide an overview of the sampling methods. Detailed procedures can be found in sources on more advanced research methodology.

Simple Random Sampling

In this method, the required number of sampling units is selected at random from the population in such a manner that each population element has an equal chance (probability) of being selected for the sample. Each choice of a sampling unit must be independent of all other choices. One of the most acceptable methods for selecting a simple random sample is to use a table of random numbers, which can be found in a statistics textbook. The numbers in a random-number table have been generated in such a way that there is no sequencing pattern. The same probability exists that

Table 6-2. Excerpt from a Table of Random Numbers

57	87	89	93	27	86	05	14	21	98
04	67	95	16	47	11	37	31	34	21
87	22	50	14	55	00	34	33	21	24
47	14	30	62	50	67	96	51	49	40
43	80	44	48	62	90	52	60	28	86
51	92	99	77	98	26	64	77	32	29
20	34	47	55	69	81	45	58	72	83
83	80	73	19	77	80	33	14	76	93
40	93	76	82	83	55	52	48	67	21
15	87	46	87	92	06	03	21	27	71
07	68	15	05	64	84	59	73	39	87

any digit will follow any other digit, and each selection was an independent choice.

To obtain a simple random sample, first list each of the population elements, then assign consecutive numbers to each of these elements. Then, referring to a table of random numbers (Table 6-2), arbitrarily start at any point in the table and proceed in any direction to identify enough tabled numbers to associate with the population elements until the desired sample has been selected.

Rather than using a table of random numbers, it is also possible to select a simple random sample by drawing numbers from a box. The names of the target population elements are written on pieces of paper which are then folded, placed in a container, and mixed well. The first name chosen is assigned to the sample, but because the probability associated with subsequent choices is not constant, the slip should be replaced in the container each time a name is selected in order to approach random selection more fully. This procedure, called *sampling with replacement,* is not as rigorous as using a table of random numbers in that each choice of a sampling unit is not independent of all other choices; once a unit is chosen, it will not be included in the sample again.

One of the problems in using simple random sampling is the difficulty of obtaining or compiling a list of each of the population elements, either because they are not known or because, for a large population, the listing proves prohibitively long.

Stratified Random Sampling

Stratified random sampling is a variation of the simple random sample. The population is divided into two or more strata or groups with different categories of a characteristic. A simple random sample is then taken from each group. This procedure is used when the composition of the population is known with respect to some characteristic or characteristics. The variables (characteristics) chosen to stratify the population must be important to the study. For example, a population of 500 human elements may be stratified on the basis of sex. Then one-half of the sampling units may be chosen from the female category and the other half from the male category by simple random sampling. This assures that the sample will consist of equal allocations from each population stratum. A population may be divided into other strata or categories, such as age, educational background, occupation, and so on.

The purpose of selecting random samples—either simple or stratified—is to permit the investigator to use appropriate inferential statistical procedures. These depend on random selection and allow the investigator to make generalizations from the sample results to the study population.

Cluster Sampling

Cluster sampling, also known as multistage sampling, is used in large-scale studies in which the population is geographically spread out. The primary sampling unit is the cluster, which consists of groups, rather than individuals, all of whom have the same characteristic. A cluster could consist of nursing homes, hospitals, or schools of nursing as the primary sampling units. For example, if the primary sampling unit is a group of hospitals, in subsequent sampling stages a random sample of the various nursing units in each hospital could be taken; then the next (cluster) stage could sample the patients on whom the actual measurements are needed for the study [3]. Cluster sampling has the advantage of convenience and involves less time and money than large-scale studies while retaining the advantages of probability sampling.

The term *systematic sampling* is used to refer to the selection of sampling units by taking every kth name on a population list, such as every fourth name listed on a hospital census sheet. Systematic sampling is considered a method of probability sampling *only if* the population list is randomly ordered (no pattern in the listing) and each population element has a known probability of being included in the sample.

Nonprobability Sampling Methods

In nonprobability sampling, the investigator has no ability to estimate the probability that each element of the population will be included in the sample. Major methods of nonprobability sampling include (1) *accidental sampling,* (2) *purposive sampling,* and (3) *quota sampling.*

Accidental Sampling

This method of sampling, *accidental sampling,* is also called *convenience sampling.* The sampling units are selected simply because they are available: They are in the right place at the right time for the investigator's purposes. For example, in the investigation of an emergency care facility during the night hours, the investigator selected an accidental sample consisting of any veteran presenting him or herself to the emergency facility for medical problems between the hours of midnight and 6:00 A.M. during a 1-month period [4]. Many nursing studies use accidental sampling because of the availability of already existing population groups.

Purposive Sampling

Purposive sampling is also called *judgment sampling*. The investigator establishes certain criteria felt to be representative of the target population and deliberately selects sampling units according to those criteria. For example, in investigating the characteristics of undergraduate nursing students most likely to succeed in graduate programs, the investigator might ask persons who are knowledgeable regarding nursing education to select the actual students for the study.

Quota Sampling

Quota sampling is much like accidental sampling, but certain controls are established so that the sample size does not become overloaded with subjects having certain characteristics. The investigator specifies a percentage for the inclusion of each characteristic in each group so that it is proportionate to the characteristics of the population. For example, quota sampling may be used to ensure that males and females from certain age, ethnic, and occupational groups are represented in the sample in proportion to these characteristics in the population.

Although it is often difficult to achieve probability sampling in clinical research, both probability and nonprobability sampling have a respected place in research. The important factor in determining which sampling approach to use is consistency with the research problem and the purpose of the study.

Sample Size

In determining how many subjects to include in a quantitative study (the total n for the study), it may be feasible to collect data regarding each element of the population. More often, however, the investigator will need to sample from the target population and must decide how large a sample will produce sufficient data to fulfill the study's purpose. There are no simple rules for determining sample size. Sample size is primarily determined by the degree of precision required, the type of sampling procedure used, the homogeneity of the population, and cost and convenience factors. There are mathematical formulas and computer programs available for calculating adequate sample size. A general rule is to use as large a sample as possible within feasible constraints. The larger the number in the sample, the more likely it is to be representative of the population from which it was selected. Representativeness of the sample is an important concern:

The question of how large a sample should be is basically unanswerable, other than to say that it should be large enough to achieve representativeness. How large this is will, of course, vary from study to study. [5]

In general, the larger the sample, the more generalizable the study results. If the population is homogeneous, a smaller sample size may be adequate.

We have found the following general guidelines helpful in determining sample size:

1. A sample of 10 percent of the population is considered a minimum for descriptive studies. For smaller populations, 20 percent may be required [6]. Fifteen subjects per group is considered minimum for experimental studies. Ten to twenty subjects per group is considered the minimum for simple studies with tight experimental control [7].
2. Statistical analysis on samples of less than 10 is not recommended and samples of 30 or more are more likely to reflect a population accurately [8].

Even with these general guidelines, the investigator should bear the following in mind:

A large sample cannot correct for a faulty sampling design. The researcher should make decisions about the sample size and design based primarily on how representative of the population the sample is likely to be. [9]

In summary, the method of selecting subjects for a quantitative study must be consistent with the problem and the purpose of the study and involves identification of the target population. If sampling is indicated, the sample should be of sufficient size to be representative of the population and should provide sufficient data for analysis. The sampling approach (probability or nonprobability) must also be consistent with the research design.

Selecting the Study Subjects in Qualitative Research

Researchers may use a number of different ways to obtain a sample for a qualitative investigation. A qualitative researcher may choose to use the same sampling methodologies that a quantitative researcher would use. There are some sampling techniques, however, that qualitative researchers might use but that quantitative researchers might choose to ignore. First, the researcher may be able to use the entire population, which is especially useful when the investigator is working in a restricted area where the population is small or lives or works in a limited setting. For example, all of the staff members or patients in a small community's hospital could be used as informants during a study.

The Nominated Sample

The *nominated* or *snowball* technique of sampling is used by some researchers. Investigators using this strategy ask their investigative questions of individuals whom they believe to have useful information. They then ask the subjects to name ("nominate") other individuals who might be able to support or give additional details concerning the research question. In this manner, the initial sample of respondents determines an additional sample of potential respondents. If the investigator does not establish trust among the research subjects, especially if the subjects are engaged in activities that might be socially unacceptable, the investigation may founder on the shoals of false information and inappropriate leads. This technique may also be called "network sampling."

Purposive Sampling

Qualitative investigators may also use *purposive* or *judgmental* sampling strategies. That is, individuals are identified as knowledgeable about the subject under investigation. If the researcher wanted to know about the perceived leadership roles of head nurses in a major hospital, for example, the main group of individuals interviewed and observed would be head nurses. Other individuals might also be interviewed and observed to provide confirmation or validation for the researcher.

Voluntary Sampling

A researcher may also issue a request for volunteers to give information. Such a request might be given through an organization such as the Red Cross (e.g., for a study of couples in prenatal or neonatal classes) or through solicitation by advertisements in newspapers or other journals. However, the investigator's data may be biased because those individuals who did not choose to volunteer might have provided data that would have either expanded or contradicted the information obtained from the volunteering subjects.

Stating the Assumptions of the Study

An assumption is a statement whose correctness or validity is taken for granted. Assumptions may be so self-evident as to require no further testing, they may be based on theories applicable to the study topic, or they may be based on previous research findings [10]. In most studies, assumptions are implied by the investigator and need not be stated explicitly. If they are significant enough to affect the study's course or outcome, the investigator should state these assumptions explicitly so that others may evaluate their effect on the study.

Stating the Limitations of the Study

The limitations of a quantitative study are restrictions that may affect the investigator's ability to generalize the study results but over which the investigator has no control. Although all studies are limited in some way, limitations in quantitative studies are usually related to the use of small, unrepresentative samples and inadequate methodology. Important limitations should be stated, both in the research proposal and in the research report, to allow the reader to judge their effect on the study. Often, qualitative researchers may not be able to state limitations prior to the study. The limitations may not be known until the qualitative researcher is in place and gathering the data.

The Workbook Activities are designed to help you evaluate your understanding of principles and procedures of data collection.

References

1. Field, P. A., and J. M. Morse. 1985. *Nursing Research: The Application of Qualitative Approaches.* Rockville, MD: Aspen, p. 139.
2. Abdellah, Faye, and Eugene Levine. 1979. *Better Patient Care through Nursing Research,* 2nd ed. New York: Macmillan, p. 152.
3. Ibid., p. 329.
4. Fiero, J. 1992. "Patients' Use of an Emergency Care Facility During the Night Hours: A Descriptive Study." In P. Dempsey and A. Dempsey. *Nursing Research with Basic Statistical Applications.* Boston: Jones and Bartlett, pp. 203–217.
5. Fox, David J. 1982. *Fundamentals of Research in Nursing,* 4th ed. New York: Appleton-Century-Crofts, p. 287.
6. Gay, L. R. 1992. *Educational Research: Competencies for Analysis and Application,* 4th ed. New York: Macmillan, p. 137.
7. Roscoe, J. T. 1975. *Fundamental Research Statistics for the Behavioral Sciences,* 2nd ed. New York: Holt, Rinehart and Winston, p. 184.
8. Ibid., p. 184.
9. Polit, D., and B. Hungler. 1992. *Nursing Research: Principles and Methods,* 4th ed. Philadelphia: J. B. Lippincott, p. 266.
10. Abdellah and Levine, *Better Patient Care,* p. 145.

Bibliography and Suggested Readings

Abdellah, F., and E. Levine. 1979. *Better Patient Care through Nursing Research,* 2nd ed. New York: Macmillan.

Brink, P. J., and M. Wood. 1994. *Basic Steps in Nursing Research.* Boston: Jones and Bartlett.

Burns, N., and S. K. Grove. 1995. *Understanding Nursing Research.* Philadelphia: W. B. Saunders.

Burns, N., and S. K. Grove. 1987. Philadelphia: W. B. Saunders.

Dempsey, P., and A. Dempsey. 1992. *Nursing Research with Basic Statistical Applications.* Boston: Jones and Bartlett.

Dobbert, M. L. 1982. *Ethnographic Research.* New York: Praeger.

Field, P. A., and J. M. Morse. 1985. *Nursing Research: The Application of Qualitative Approaches.* Rockville, MD: Aspen.

Fiero, J. 1992. "Patients' Use of an Emergency Care Facility During the Night Hours: A Descriptive Study." In P. Dempsey and A. Dempsey. *Nursing Research with Basic Statistical Applications.* Boston: Jones and Bartlett, pp. 203–217.

Ford, J. 1975. *Paradigms and Fairy Tales.* London: Routledge and Kegan Paul.

Fox, D. 1982. *Fundamentals of Research in Nursing,* 4th ed. New York: Appleton-Century-Crofts.

Gay, L. R. 1987. *Educational Research: Competencies for Analysis and Application,* 3rd ed. Columbus, OH: Charles E. Merrill.

Goetz, J. P., and M. D. LeCompte. 1984. *Ethnography and Qualitative Design in Educational Research.* Orlando, FL: Academic Press.

Halley, S., and S. Cummings. 1988. *Designing Clinical Research: An Epidemiological Approach.* Baltimore, MD: Williams and Wilkins.

Hopkins, C. D. 1976. *Educational Research: A Structure for Inquiry.* Columbus, OH: Charles E. Merrill.

Kidder, L., C. M. Judd, and E. R. Smith. 1986. *Research Methods in Social Relations,* 5th ed. New York: Holt, Rinehart and Winston.

Morse, J. 1989. *Qualitative Nursing Research: A Contemporary Dialogue.* Rockville, MD: Aspen.

Polit, D., and B. Hungler. 1992. *Nursing Research Principles and Methods,* 4th ed. Philadelphia: J. B. Lippincott.

Roscoe, J. T. 1975. *Fundamental Research Statistics for the Behavioral Sciences,* 2nd ed. New York: Holt, Rinehart and Winston.

Selby-Harrington, M. L., et al. 1994. "Reporting of Instrument Validity and Reliability in Selected Clinical Nursing Journals, 1989." *Journal of Professional Nursing,* 10 (January–February): 47–56.

United Nations. 1973. *A Short Manual on Sampling, Volume II: Computer Programmes for Sampling Design.* New York: United Nations Press.

Werner, W., and G. M. Schoepfle. 1987. *Systematic Fieldwork.* Beverly Hills, CA: Sage.

7 The Historical Research Approach

Objectives

When you have finished reading this chapter you should be able to:

1. Discuss the difference between secondary and primary resources in historical research

2. List and describe several primary resources for historical research

3. Discuss how validity is determined in historical research

4. Discuss how reliability is determined in historical research

---

The Nature of Historical Research
Methodology
Secondary Data Sources
  Interpretations
  Hearsay
Primary Data Sources
  Oral History
  Life History
  Published Sources
  Diaries
  Historical Societies
  Official Minutes
  Audio and Visual Recordings
  Eyewitnesses
  Pictorial Sources
  Other Print Sources
  Physical Evidence
Computers and Historical Research
Validity and Reliability

Nursing is both a very young profession and a very old one. Even before Greek and Roman soldiers were carried home on their shields—sometimes dead and sometimes wounded—someone has always been charged with the care of the ill or injured.

Before 1859 and the Crimean War, nurses of either sex were often camp followers, prostitutes, and thieves. Florence Nightingale's heroic ministrations to the sick and wounded British soldiers helped to raise nursing to the respectability it enjoys today. However, this respectability did not come about simply as a result of Nightingale's work. Many more subtle battles have been fought against those individuals who have deeply resented the rapid changing of the traditional nursing role.

We do not wish to chronicle Nightingale's life or those of any other heroic characters of nursing. This brief introduction to the founding of modern nursing is intended to set the scene for an examination of the techniques of historical research.

The Nature of Historical Research

Historical research deals with what has happened in the past and how those events affect the present. No professional group is more in the forefront of world history than nursing. By its very nature, nursing is always where the action is. Nurses have been active in all areas of the world both in times of conflict and in times of peace, yet nursing history has tended to center around a few semimythologized individuals.

The lives and times of these individuals are important to nursing, but historical research is more than the discovery and adulation of famous individuals. Historical research covers all people and events. Historians piece together the lives of less well known and less controversial individuals to get a picture of the actual lives and times of an era. The historian uses these data to determine the impact of history on the present and occasionally tries to predict the future on the basis of this knowledge.

Methodology

Essentially, the historian follows the same kind of research format as any other researcher. First, the problem to be investigated must be selected and formulated within the context of existing knowledge and theory. For a historical research study, a hypothesis may be tested. Like any other researcher, the historical researcher must be particularly careful in gathering and interpreting data and in drawing conclusions based on those data. Historical research lends itself to the acceptance of evidence that is hard to verify. The careful researcher must do the utmost to corroborate data and to demonstrate the reliability and validity of the data. Data sources available to the historical researcher fall into two categories, secondary and primary.

Secondary Data Sources

Secondary sources are the least trustworthy. They are of two basic types: (1) interpretations by someone else of documented data and (2) hearsay.

Interpretations

The use of interpretations by someone else of documented data is fraught with peril. Historical researchers depend on another person's private frame of reference for information. This means that their interpretations may or may not be totally correct. Just as a television commercial can tell you that almost 50 percent of the people polled preferred one product over another product (leaving out the fact that *more* than 50 percent did not prefer this product), so, too, the historical researcher may choose to emphasize those facts and data that fit his or her hypothesis. This is not good research, but it does exist and can lead to further misinterpretation of data. In fact, the farther a researcher is from the original historical data, the greater the chance of misinterpretation. It is crucial that the historical researcher go back to the original sources whenever possible. The bibliography and footnotes of secondary sources often lead to primary sources, which can then be checked for accuracy of interpretation and used for gathering additional data. No secondary source, no matter how carefully prepared, can provide a total interpretation of all the data. All historians must select and interpret from a variety of sources.

Hearsay

The second, and possibly the most naive, secondary source is hearsay evidence. Hearsay is simply what people think they heard or, even worse, the extension of unproved rumors and gossip. We all know how easy it is to misinterpret and pass along incorrect information. The classic example is the game called "telephone," in which a group of people sit in a circle and one person starts by whispering a sentence or phrase to the next person. The message is then passed around the circle until it comes back to its original source. It is always interesting to discover how the message has changed along the way. Historical researchers must be extremely careful when dealing with hearsay data. It may be old and valuable or it may totally misrepresent the facts. Every effort must be made to corroborate any piece of hearsay data and to place it into proper historical perspective.

Primary Data Sources

Primary data are of far greater value and importance to the historian than secondary data. Primary data can be found in many forms and in many places.

Oral History

One of the most exciting current historical movements is called *oral history*. Electronic devices, such as the audio- or videotape recorder, have made it possible to record the remembrances of older members of the professional community, thus providing records of what took place in past times and in specific places. These older people are invaluable resources and, as they die, their information is lost forever.

Essentially, oral historians transcribe the tapes and reproduce the conversations in writing. These data must be carefully screened, but they do provide an important *primary source*. The oral historian should plan a list of questions for the interviewee to help start the conversation off and to keep it on the subject. The historian should also get permission to reproduce this information. Many things may be said off the record, but they are of no value to the historian. Only evidence for the record can be utilized.

Life History

Life histories or career histories are an extension of the oral history technique. The proposal in Appendix A is designed to elicit a career history of one individual who had a significant impact on the field of nursing.

When researchers gather life or career histories from several individuals who are contemporaries, the researchers can go beyond discussing the lives of the individuals and begin to interpret and discuss the whole cultural milieu in which these individuals worked and lived. For example, if one source says that a certain organization or individual was helpful in developing his or her career, the information is useful only insofar as it relates to that individual. But if a number of individuals name the same organization or individual as influential, the researcher can then draw a broader conclusion.

Published Sources

Published sources are valuable to the historical researcher. There is an increasing trend to store old newspapers, journals, magazines, and other published material on one of the various microform sources. This means that the historical researcher does not have to travel great distances to get to the few remaining copies of the material. Rather, a microform copy can be ordered from the producer and reviewed by using a microform reader, which is readily available in most college and university libraries and in an increasing number of public libraries. The listings available can be found in *Microforms in Print.*

Other published sources available are the original documents themselves. Many items of interest to nurses and nursing can be found in popular literature either in the form of articles about nurses and nursing or as fictional representations of nurses and their role. Early items are indexed in *Poole's Index* and the *Readers' Guide to Periodical Literature.* Neither of these may contain a complete listing, but both will aid in the library search.

Government documents are an excellent source for the historical researcher. Many governments have compiled enormous quantities of official records and documents. In addition to the national government, state and local governments also abound with records. Many source data have been lost over the years as county courthouses and other document repositories have burned accidentally. Yet many other promising avenues of research are open to the researcher who is not afraid of the dust and grime usually found in these seldom-used sources.

Diaries

Diaries can provide an invaluable source of documentation. These are often handed down from generation to generation in a family; the researcher must locate families who still have these documents in their possession and are willing to share their intimate contents. Diary research requires judicious questioning and a substantial amount of careful exploration.

Historical Societies

Often, there will be a local historical group that a researcher can contact. These groups are justifiably proud of the community's history and can provide access to many documents and to individuals with specific knowledge. All of this can be invaluable to an outside researcher.

Official Minutes

Obviously, the availability of minutes and records of meetings is important. It is wise to remember, however, that the minutes of meetings usually reflect an abridged version of what really happened. Acrimonious debate or nonvoted issues often are not shown in minutes. Remember, each legislator has the privilege of editing what he or she has said on the floor of the U.S. House or Senate before such speeches are finally placed in the *Congressional Record.* Thus, the speeches we read are not necessarily verbatim reports of what was actually said.

Audio and Visual Recordings

Current technology has made a great deal of audio and visual source materials available. Records, tape and wire recordings, and film and videotapes all provide invaluable historical insight. Much of this material may be rare and hard to obtain. Locating appropriate sources can be a tedious yet fascinating job.

Eyewitnesses

Eyewitness accounts are always useful. Written eyewitness accounts may be found in newspapers, as oral history, or in diaries. It is crucial that eyewitness accounts receive corroboration from other sources because such accounts may report only a small part of the whole.

Pictorial Sources

Still photographs and other pictorial sources, such as sketches, are extremely valuable items. Certainly Matthew Brady and the other photographers of the American Civil War provided visual portraits of times and places that could only be imagined if we had nothing more than the written documents. Again, even as personal diaries are rich resources, so are family picture albums. They can be used to find out a great deal about the history of a group of people in any locality.

Other Print Sources

Other valid source materials for historical research might be old telephone books and directories, catalogs of local businesses and national concerns, and accounting books and bank records.

Physical Evidence

Do not ignore physical evidence of change throughout the years. For example, there have been many alterations in the various types of equipment used by nurses. Many of the products of technical change that have been added to the repertoire of nursing can be used as source materials for historical research.

Computers and Historical Research

Like other researchers, historical researchers are turning more and more to the computer for help. In some instances, the computer can be used to locate and reprint historical documents. Some historians have examined numerical data statistically and have drawn conclusions about the conditions of individuals in a given historical period. This use of statistical methodology is called *cliometrics*. Sometimes this method has been used to demonstrate that certain cherished ideas were incorrect. As a consequence, the use of the computer in historical research is somewhat controversial.

Validity and Reliability

In all cases, the historical researcher must question the reliability and validity of sources by applying both *internal* and *external* criticism to the written document. External criticism deals with the validity of the document: Is it really what it purports to be? Internal criticism deals with the reliability or accuracy of the information. Some of the questions that should be asked include: Is this document consistent with other documents written by this person? Does it have the same style? Does the style match the style of the time? Are the spelling and handwriting consistent with the time? Is what the document saying true? It is very easy to fool a naive researcher with manufactured documents like the so-called Hitler diaries. Caution must be the watchword when dealing with historical material.

In this chapter we discussed the principles and techniques of historical research. Discovering the past through careful documentation can provide many important insights into the present.

Bibliography and Suggested Readings

Austen, A. L. 1957. *History of Nursing Sourcebook.* New York: G. P. Putnam's Sons.

Baly, M. 1986. *Florence Nightingale and the Nursing Legacy.* London: Routledge, Chapman and Hall.

Benjamin, J. R. 1975. *A Student's Guide to History.* New York: St. Martin's Press.

Bogue, A. G. 1983. *Clio and the Bitch Goddess: Quantification in American Political History.* Beverly Hills, CA: Sage.

Christy, T. E. 1975. "The Methodology of Historical Research." *Nursing Research,* 24 (May–June): 189–192.

Clark, G. 1969. *Guide for Research Students Working on Historical Subjects,* 2nd ed. London: Cambridge University Press.

Dingwall, R., and C. W. Rafferty. 1988. *An Introduction to the Social History of Nursing.* London: Routledge.

Dock, L. L. 1912. *A History of Nursing.* New York: G. P. Putnam's Sons.

Dock, L. L., and I. Stewart. 1920. *A Short History of Nursing.* New York: G. P. Putnam's Sons.

Donahue, M. P. 1985. *Nursing: The Finest Art, an Illustrated History.* St. Louis: Mosby.

Fairman, Julie A. 1987. "Sources and References for Research in Nursing History." *Nursing Research,* 36 (January–February): 56–59.

Hawkins, J. W. 1987. *The Historical Evolution of Theories and Conceptual Models for Nursing.* Educational Resources Information Center (ERIC) ED 284969.

History of American Nursing Series. New York: Garland Press.

Interagency Council on Library Sources for Nursing. 1989. *Guide to Archival Sources in Nursing.* West Long Branch, NJ: The Interagency Council.

Jones, A. H., Ed. 1987. *Images of Nurses: Perspectives from History, Art and Literature.* Philadelphia: University of Pennsylvania Press.

Kalish, P. A., and B. J. Kalish. 1986. *The Advance of American Nursing,* 2nd ed. Boston: Little, Brown.

Lagermann, E. C., Ed. 1983. *Nursing History: New Perspectives, New Possibilities.* New York: Teachers College, Columbia University.

Moore, J. 1988. *A Zeal for Responsibility.* Athens: University of Georgia.

Rice, M. H., and W. M. Stallings. 1986. *Florence Nightingale, Statistician: Implications for Teachers of Educational Research.* Educational Resources Information Center (ERIC) ED 269452.

Roberts, M. M. 1954. *American Nursing: History and Interpretation.* New York: Macmillan.

Rosenberg, C. 1987. "Clio and Caring: An Agenda for American Historians and Nursing." *Nursing Research,* 36 (January–February): 67–68.

8 The Descriptive Research Approach

Objectives

When you have finished this chapter you should be able to:

1. Describe several descriptive research techniques

2. Develop a questionnaire with multiple-choice responses

3. Develop a rating scale

4. Develop a questionnaire for a structured interview

5. Describe and compare qualitative research approaches

The Nature of Descriptive Research
Descriptive Research Techniques
　Electrical and Mechanical Devices to Measure Physiologic Responses
　Questionnaires
　Interviews
　Rating Scales
　Content Analysis
　Use of Available Data
　Unobtrusive Measures
　Nonwritten Records
　Proxemics and Kinesics
　Case Studies
　Psychological and Projective Tests
　Sociometrics
　Delphi Technique
　Observation
Qualitative Strategies for Descriptive Research
　Phenomenology
　Ethnography
　Grounded Theory
Summary

The material covered in this chapter explores the descriptive research approach and the techniques and tools most frequently used to gather data needed to study present conditions.

The Nature of Descriptive Research

The *descriptive research approach* describes what now exists, but the term is not completely appropriate. Description is also involved in the other two approaches: *Historical research* describes the past, and *experimental research* describes what happens to selected variables in order to predict what will happen as other variables are manipulated by the investigator. *Descriptive research* is used here to refer to research questions based on the present state of affairs and yields both quantitative and qualitative data. Such research may generate new knowledge beyond the study's specific subjects or elements.

Descriptive Research Techniques

The techniques for gathering data about present conditions are intended to provide information that can be analyzed either quantitatively or qualitatively. The techniques most often used to study present conditions, which can be used to study contrasts (differences), comparisons (likenesses), and relationships, include the following:

1. Electrical and mechanical devices
2. Questionnaires
3. Interviews
4. Rating scales
5. Content analysis
6. Use of available data
7. Unobtrusive measures
8. Nonwritten records
9. Proxemics and kinesics
10. Case studies
11. Psychological and projective tests
12. Sociometrics
13. Delphi technique
14. Observation
15. Phenomenology
16. Ethnography
17. Grounded theory

Each of these techniques will be discussed in greater detail in the following pages.

Electrical and Mechanical Devices to Measure Physiologic Responses

By its very nature, nursing research lends itself to the use of highly accurate physiologic measurements. There are an increasing number of sophisticated measuring devices available to determine physiologic responses. Of course, the classic mechanical devices, such as the sphygmomanometer and the stethoscope, have been developed and refined over many years. In addition, many electronic devices, such as the electrocardiograph, the electroencephalograph, and other instruments, are now available.

As in all research dealing with human subjects, when mechanical or electrical devices are used, researchers have the ethical responsibility to obtain informed consent and to explain the purpose of any device that is used to determine patients' responses. It is extremely frightening to be attached to a mechanical device of some kind without knowing why.

Questionnaires

The term *survey research* is often used to refer to the collection of data about present conditions directly from the study subjects. The most common techniques for survey research are the questionnaire and the interview.

A *questionnaire* is a paper-and-pencil instrument completed by the study subjects themselves. In survey research, the questionnaire is often mailed to the respondents, although it might be administered face to face. An *opinionnaire* is a questionnaire designed to elicit the subjects' opinions. The term *interview* refers to verbal questioning of respondents by the investigator in order to collect data. The interview may be conducted either face to face or by telephone.

Nursing researchers have developed many survey instruments—primarily questionnaires—over the years. The respondents may be nurses, patients, patients' relatives, or doctors, among many alternatives. These survey instruments have been designed to examine attitudes, opinions, feelings, and facts concerning certain areas of nursing. Such instruments can accurately reflect these opinions, feelings, and facts only if they are well developed, well administered, and carefully interpreted.

Longitudinal Studies

Some investigators with long-term interests use the same measuring instrument repeatedly in order to determine responses on a topic and pinpoint trends and issues. Such studies, known as *longitudinal studies,* are designed to collect data from the same people at regularly stated intervals, ranging from a few days to weeks, months, or even years.

Cross-Sectional Studies

The vast majority of surveys, however, are one-time *cross-sectional studies*. They study certain aspects of responses of individuals at a certain point in time and are seldom, if ever, conducted again. This is unfortunate because it leads to a proliferation of data-gathering instruments, some of which may not be very good. In addition, the lack of repeated measurement over time prevents the analysis of trends concerning various issues.

Researchers use surveys to gather information from a representative sample of a population. The researcher can specify the location of the population, such as all patients admitted to the emergency room of hospital XYZ, or only those patients admitted to the emergency room between the hours of noon and midnight. Such specificity allows for the use of probability sampling techniques; with good statistical analysis, generalizations can be drawn about the whole population. As discussed in Chapter 6, the researcher must take care to ensure an accurate description of the target population as well as the sample. Whether the population is 24- to 27-year-old postpartum mothers with female infants or any other of the large number of possible combinations, the best research defines specifically who will be surveyed.

With these ideas in mind, we will now describe the steps in designing and carrying out survey research using questionnaires.

Development and Administration

First, as with any research study, an appropriate research question or problem must be established. The problem statement and the purpose of the study should guide the selection of an appropriate survey research design and the choice of a measuring instrument that meets the criteria of validity, reliability, and usability, as discussed in Chapter 6. The following principles apply to self-developed questionnaires constructed by the investigator for a specific study.

In constructing a questionnaire, care must be exercised so that the items will allow the respondents to provide the information that relates to the study problem and to the purpose of the study. The theoretical or conceptual framework should provide the rationale for the development of the questionnaire.

Questionnaires are constructed to be either open-ended or closed. Open-ended questionnaires allow the respondents a variety of ways to answer questions and permit the researcher to make inferences from the responses to the questions. Closed questionnaires allow for certain structured answers—"yes," "no," or a limited selection of choices. Because most survey researchers want to expedite the coding of data and eliminate ambiguity, they usually opt for a closed questionnaire.

The questionnaire must be clear and unambiguous. We tend to assume that people understand what we are talking about, but the naive respondent may not have the same frame of reference as the researcher. The question "Are the chickens ready to eat?" is a good example of the ambiguous use of our language. Any question that could have multiple interpretations should also be avoided.

The wording of questions should be concise. Avoid asking a wordy question when a brief one will do. Respondents not familiar with the vocabulary will not give accurate or valid answers. At the same time, respect the respondent's intelligence. This means walking a fine line. The more confusion or mistrust the instrument causes, the less chance there will be that the respondent will return the questionnaire.

Keep the questionnaire as simple and short as possible. There is something very threatening about an instrument with many pages and a multiplicity of choices. The shorter the instrument (within reason), the more likely it will be completed and returned. Be sure to put relatively simple questions at the beginning of the instrument, allowing the respondent to succeed and be reinforced to continue.

Provide cross-check questions in order to be sure that the respondent is answering consistently. Rewording the same question and asking it again, either positively or negatively, is a good way to provide this insurance, but questions should be sufficiently separated so that the subject will not see through this technique.

Finally, careful development of the instructions for the respondent involves a clear statement of what you want the respondent to do. Validity and reliability must be determined by using any one of the techniques described in Chapter 6. We strongly recommend that a pretest of the questionnaire be conducted in order to correct any problem with the questionnaire before it is administered to the study subjects.

Researchers should probably spend more time formulating their questionnaires than they do analyzing their research data. Well-constructed questionnaires allow for relatively easy interpretation and analysis. Poorly developed questionnaires may cost more in time and effort and prevent the investigator from achieving the purpose of the study.

Mailed questionnaires are answered in much larger numbers if a self-addressed, stamped envelope is included with each questionnaire. Most people are willing to respond but unwilling to subsidize the researcher. If a follow-up letter is sent, it may be wise to send yet another self-addressed, stamped envelope and questionnaire. Granted, this may add to the researcher's expenditures, but all research should be planned to include the total cost of all items.

Cover letters are important and should include the following items:

1. Name of the researcher
2. Address of the researcher
3. Purpose of the study
4. Approximate length of time required to fill out the questionnaire
5. A statement safeguarding the confidentiality of the responses
6. Any other information the researcher feels is important

When using a mailed questionnaire, the investigator should allow a specific amount of time to elapse after the survey instrument has been mailed and should determine an acceptable percentage of responses to be obtained. This is necessary because there are many reasons for nonresponses to any survey, especially if the survey instrument is mailed. Any investigator who expects a 100 percent response will probably never draw any conclusions from the study.

Interviews

There are two basic kinds of interviewing techniques: structured and unstructured. In the *structured interview* the interviewer has a list of prepared questions that the researcher believes will provide a format for the respondent's answers concerning the researcher's project—for example, (1) How friendly do the nurses in ZZZ hospital seem to be? (2) Why do you answer as you do? The interviewer thus guides the respondent to determine what information is elicited and then records the answers.

An *unstructured interview* is more like a conversation. Here the researcher has a general framework of questions to elicit answers concerning the information sought, but uses the respondent's answers to enlarge upon the topic and to ask additional questions. The topics flow from the conversation's progress, and there is no set pattern or ordering of the categories that the researcher is exploring. Unstructured interviews take more time than structured interviews. The researcher must search the record of responses in order to categorize and organize the data elicited.

It is always the researcher's responsibility to provide adequate training for the interviewers who may be assisting in the collection of the study data. Face-to-face interviewers must be nonthreatening to the respondent. Certain styles of dress and manners may be appropriate in one setting but not in another. Each interviewer must gain rapport and trust with the respondent. Interviewers should be trained to remain neutral when eliciting answers to the survey instrument. Many people will give the answer that they think the interviewer wants to hear rather than what they really believe. Interviewers who encourage such responses, whether overtly or unconsciously, cannot gather valid data.

A pilot or preliminary study is extremely valuable as a part of the training process. Debriefing after a few interviews allows the interviewers to point out flaws not initially discovered in the interview schedules and coding sheets. It also provides for a check on interviewing techniques.

Remember, too, that the interviewer will be doing two separate things during the course of the interview. First, the questions or statements must be given to the respondent and the appropriate response elicited. Second, the interviewer must mark a coded response sheet or record what the respondent says. Obviously, the statements on the response sheet must be organized carefully so that the interviewer can perform these tasks with a minimum of problems. If it is physically difficult to code the responses, the chance of error increases significantly.

It is usually easier to gain interviews if the interviewers have official sanction. When planning to interview members of a community, for example, the researcher might contact local city officials. Frequently they will be willing to provide a letter, badge, or other symbol of official recognition, which gives interviewers easier access to study subjects. It is helpful to remember that in a small community news travels fast. If the interviewing techniques are displeasing, potential respondents may reject the interviewers on the basis of what they have heard from others in the community.

Telephone interviewers should also be selected with care. Respondents visualize the individual on the other end of the line, so the interviewer should have a pleasing telephone voice and should have practiced using the survey instrument a number of times before actually talking to potential respondents.

It is noteworthy that people seem increasingly resistant to responding to telephone surveys. This may be due to a number of factors. First, with the increasing popularity of telephone surveys, individuals find that their time is being demanded more frequently. Second, there have been frequent misrepresentations by telephone solicitors who claim to be conducting a survey but are actually selling a product. Finally, more and more people have come to resent intrusion into their privacy.

Respondents should be given an opportunity to receive the results of the study. After being a respondent in any survey, the individual has an interest in finding out what came about as a result of the study. The offer to provide a summary of the study's results will often entice individuals who might not otherwise participate or respond. Be sure to keep your word; failure to provide the promised information may ruin future research possibilities both for yourself and for others.

Rating Scales

A *rating scale* is a type of data-collecting instrument that allows the respondents to place their feelings or attitudes on a scale. For example:

How would you rate the nursing care in this hospital?

Very good ____:____:____:____:____:____ Very poor
Please check the appropriate blank.

The number of response options on rating scales may vary considerably. Although five options occur most frequently, and this appears to be the minimum acceptable number, six, seven, or eight options can also be presented. The *Likert Scale* is a rating scale in which each statement usually has five possible responses: strongly agree, agree, uncertain, disagree, strongly disagree. A Likert-type scale may have more or fewer response choices, however.

There is a definite advantage in using even-numbered scales. These are called *forced choice* scales. When given an odd number of choices, subjects may respond to the middle choice and thus appear to be neutral, choosing neither high nor low ratings. If a scale has an even number of options, the subject must respond with a high or low ranking or rating. Given the previous question, the forced choice scale compels the respondent to like or dislike the nursing care.

The nursing care in this hospital is:

Very good ____:____:____:____:____:____ Very poor

The scale might similarly have been written:

The nursing care in this hospital is very good.
VSA   SA   A   D   SD   VSD

The responses stand for very strongly agree, strongly agree, agree, disagree, strongly disagree, very strongly disagree, respectively. In this instance the respondent would probably be asked to circle the appropriate response.

Sometimes, if the sample size is small, adequate statistical analysis cannot be done. Forced choice scales allow for the collapsing of cells (categories of data), for dichotomization, or for bringing cells together in statistically valid groups. Neutral responses might otherwise have to be discarded or divided, giving an unclear picture of the respondents' feelings or attitudes.

Respondents may be asked to *rank order* their responses from the most important to the least important. This technique can be very effective. If the rank order list is too long, however, the subjects may have trouble keeping the whole list in mind. For example:

Nurses should be capable of participating in research. The following is a list of settings in which nursing research can be carried out. Please rank each in order of importance as a setting for nursing research by placing a "6" by the most important, a "5" by the second most important, and so on down to number "1" (least important).

( ) hospital
( ) community health center
( ) visiting nurses association
( ) hospice
( ) day care center
( ) home health agency

A type of rating scale that has had a great deal of interest and success is called the *semantic differential scale*. This tool consists of a list of bipolar adjectives that may describe a setting, object, profession, or any other variable. For example, if we want to determine how people from different cultural and ethnic backgrounds perceive hospitals, we might construct the following:

Below is a checklist of words that describe a hospital. Please place a check mark in the space that best shows how you feel about hospitals. Be sure to place a check mark on each line.

Hospitals

Good___:___:___:___:___:___:___Bad
Busy___:___:___:___:___:___:___Quiet
Warm___:___:___:___:___:___:___Cold
Clean___:___:___:___:___:___:___Dirty

Various analytical techniques can be applied to the items in a semantic differential scale to determine if different subjects perceive the hospital setting in different ways.

Multiple-choice questions have long been a staple of examinations. They may also be used for eliciting research data. For example:

Place a circle around the letter of the response that most accurately reflects your point of view about the following items:

1. People have strong feelings about a national health care program. Which of the following statements best represents your attitude toward national health care?
   a. National health care will cost too much to be practical and should be avoided.

  b. National health care is the only way to provide adequate health care for all people.

  c. National health care should be limited to catastrophic illnesses.

  d. National health care would subvert our free enterprise system.

Note that in this instance respondents may not agree with any of the choices. Care must be exercised in developing this kind of instrument so that experimenter bias does not creep in through the use of slanted questions.

Content Analysis

Up to this point we have been discussing closed or structured measuring instruments: instruments that allow the respondent few or no alternatives in their responses. Frequently, as you probably have experienced, there is a feeling or response of "yes, but . . ." The respondents would like to qualify their answers or provide reasons for them. Open-ended measuring instruments allow respondents to explain why they respond in a particular manner. For example:

> Do you believe that the hospital staff should be differentiated by the color of their uniforms—blue for RNs, green for aides, yellow for LPNs, etc.? Please explain your answer.

This type of instrument lends itself to *content analysis.* The researcher examines the responses to determine the frequently cited reasons, compares adjective use between different groups, or uses one of a large number of potential analytical techniques. Obviously, with large samples and many responses, this technique can become tedious. Careful analysis of responses and documents can reveal a great deal that might otherwise be lost if closed or structured measuring instruments were used.

Use of Available Data

The increasing number of nursing studies over the years has created a large pool of *available data.* Studies that give complete reports of the number of respondents and their responses can be reanalyzed using other statistical tools to determine if the original conclusions were accurate. As a result of technologic advances, these tools are often more sophisticated than those available to the original reseacher. Furthermore, comparisons and contrasts can be made between past and current study responses. For example, a renewed interest in the study of sociobiology has led to a great deal of controversy at the present time. Reanalysis of existing data from sociobiologic studies done at the beginning of the century might well be a valid research project at this time. Many such data are open to reinterpretation based on current knowledge and techniques.

Other available data sources include the reports of the large number of specialized statistic-gathering organizations, census tract reports, licensing bureau reports, and the reports of other organizations that gather and report data about people or groups of people. For example, a college placement service might have information about the type and level of employment held by nursing graduates. This might lead to conclusions about the success of the school in educating its students and might also point out strengths and weaknesses.

Unobtrusive Measures

Over the years, an increasing number of studies have used *unobtrusive measures*. The researcher decides what needs to be measured and then determines how to measure it without direct intervention. A time-honored way to measure the most popular exhibits in a museum would be to determine the dirtiest display cases at the end of the day; this is done on the assumption that the more people who touch or press their noses against a display case, the dirtier it will be. Over a period of time, certain exhibits would show the most consistent usage [1].

Anxiety levels could be measured by observing the wear and tear on magazines placed in waiting rooms. Perhaps more stress is exhibited in the office of a dentist than in the waiting room of an emergency facility.

Nonwritten Records

A number of techniques are available to preserve the activities of individuals and groups in an enduring format. In the past, still photographs and pictures were used to analyze the behavior, beliefs, dress, and activities of subjects. With the advent of motion pictures, more details could be captured. Today, these techniques, as well as the technology of video- and audiotapes, can provide long-lasting records for future use and study.

Proxemics and Kinesics

Proxemics studies the use of time and space in communication. Americans, for example, often become uncomfortable when people from other countries or cultures approach and engage them in conversation. The person may be felt to be standing too close, and this makes the American nervous because his or her "body space" is being invaded. The other person is also uncomfortable, and feels that the American is being standoffish. Both individuals are right. Cultural background defines how far apart individuals should be when communicating. Nurses might design research using videotape technology to study how patients from various cultures interact and react when communicating with nurses from the same and different cultures.

Kinesics is the observation of nonverbal communication. Almost all individuals learn appropriate methods of nonverbal communication, ranging from the smiles and frowns of the very young to the posture with which one carries oneself. Again, videotapes can be used to analyze how individuals react and interact nonverbally regardless of their verbal reactions and interactions.

Case Studies

The use of *case studies* might be considered a particular methodology within the category of descriptive research techniques. Social anthropologists have long been concerned with rather large groups of individuals, especially those sharing a common culture or background. In the case study method, a general population sharing a common background is identified, but the researcher works with a limited number of individuals, ranging from one person to a large sample. (Statistical research carried out on an individual is known as *single-subject research*.) The researcher then carefully observes and documents all the activities, contacts, and other salient actions of the individual(s).

Using the case study method, a nurse might document the activities of several hospital supervisors to determine if differences in leadership styles existed in the obstetric service as opposed to the intensive care units.

Psychological and Projective Tests

Sometimes a researcher may want to determine more than surface attitudes about something. Perhaps the intent is to understand why a patient feels the way he or she does. Because it is impossible to read a person's mind, inferential instruments must be used. Consistency of responses can indicate a frame of reference, a mind-set, or a set of ideas.

Psychiatry and psychology have developed a number of instruments to determine a patient's feelings. These are called *projective tests* because the patient projects a meaning into materials that are essentially ambiguous or meaningless.

We have all heard of the Rorschach (ink blot) test. An individual is asked to look at a standard series of abstract forms (ink blots) and tell what he or she sees. Because the forms are random in shape, the subject must project or put meaning into them from his or her own beliefs or ideas. By presenting a series of these items, the researcher can draw conclusions about the subject's state of mind.

The Thematic Apperception Test (TAT) is frequently used to determine feelings and ideas. In this test subjects are shown pictures of people in ambiguous situations and asked to describe what is happening. Again, the subject must project his or her own feelings into the situation, allowing the researcher to draw conclusions about the individual.

Projective tests can be very helpful, but the researcher must interpret the responses cautiously. The very nature of the devices can lead to misunderstanding and misinterpretation. Much training is necessary before a researcher puts these devices into use.

As discussed in Chapter 6, we strongly recommend that researchers go to as many sources as possible to determine if a preexisting measuring instrument is available. Frequently, an appropriate instrument is available, with reliability and validity already established. A few hours of library search with such resources as *Mental Measurements Yearbook* or *Tests in Print* may save several weeks of development time.

Sociometrics

Sometimes a researcher wants to determine the social interaction and patterns of leadership roles in a group. This can be determined by the use of *sociometric techniques*. Essentially, the researcher structures a questionnaire to determine the most desirable or the most favorably perceived individuals in a group. Questions used in sociometrics might include the following:

1. Who is the best nurse on the unit?
2. Which nurses are the most effective? Name three.
3. Which three nurses do you like working with the best?

You may want to develop a sociogram to diagram the responses (Fig. 8-1) or you may want to develop a social matrix showing the responses in tabular form (Table 8-1). These techniques can provide some very important information about the group's informal structure, who the informal leaders are, and where the power really lies.

Delphi Technique

One survey technique that has been popular in the past few years is known as the *Delphi technique*. Named after the famous Oracle of Apollo at Delphi, the process attempts to predict what will be important to the surveyed group in the future.

The Delphi technique consists of identifying a group of experts or persons concerned with a certain area or program. Their concerns about their area or program are elicited and ranked. Once a total list of concerns has

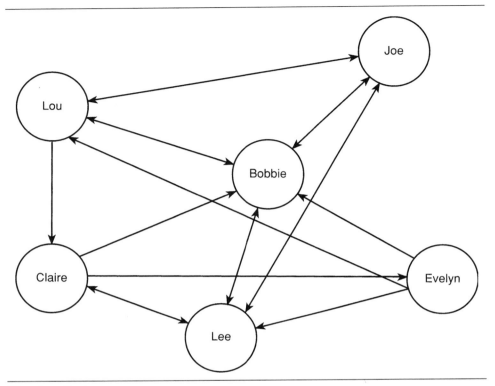

Fig. 8-1. Sociogram

Table 8-1. Social Matrix

Selectee	Selector					
	Lee	Claire	Evelyn	Lou	Joe	Bobbie
Lee	—	X	X		X	X
Claire	X	—		X		
Evelyn		X	—			
Lou			X	—	X	X
Joe	X			X	—	X
Bobbie	X	X	X	X	X	—

been acquired, it is given to the experts, who are asked to rank the items on the list in order of importance.

The responses are again tallied by the researcher and sent back to the same panel with response totals given. The panel members are then asked to rerank their responses on the basis of the total responses and their peers' evaluations. The researcher can then focus on those items considered the most important by the experts.

For example, we might use the Delphi technique to examine nurses' concerns in a community health agency by sending out the following questions to all, or a sample, of the staff nurses.

> We are attempting to determine the future goals for patient care in a community setting. Please list at least five of your major concerns about nursing service as it is currently practiced in a community setting.

As you can see, each of the respondents then has an opportunity to express concerns and predictions about the future of nursing care in the community.

After the first round of responses is returned, the researcher lists each comment—with similar comments organized into a single topic—and a questionnaire is developed. The same respondents are used in all rounds of questioning so that a letter like the following might be sent to the initial respondents.

> Several weeks ago you were asked to list your major concerns about the patient care in your community. As a result of your responses and those of your peers, we have been able to develop the following list of concerns. We would now like you to rate these concerns on a scale of 1 to 5, with 1 being of little importance and 5 being of great importance.

1. Patient loads are too large for adequate care to be given.

1 2 3 4 5

2. Patients are unable to get additional care from other community agencies.

1 2 3 4 5

After the subjects respond to this questionnaire, the researcher then calculates how each response was evaluated by determining the percentages of the total responses in each category. For instance, the group sampled on the question concerning patient loads might have responded 60 percent 5's, 20 percent 4's, and 20 percent 3's. Another survey is then sent to the respondents with a letter that might read like this:

> You and your colleagues have responded to a series of questions concerning nursing care in your community. Each of you was asked to rank a list of questions as to their importance. Based on your responses, the questions were rated by the percentages in the categories which you see below. Please rate the questions as to their importance again, based on your own beliefs and your knowledge of your peers' responses.

At this point, the subjects may also be supplied with their own previous responses. The subjects then respond and rate the questions as to their relative importance. The researcher reevaluates the scale and determines which items are now considered the most important by the respondents. The researcher then identifies the main areas of concern and makes recommendations.

The Delphi technique has the advantage of identifying the group's major concerns and can be used to make recommendations to alleviate these concerns. It also allows an organization to focus on and take direction toward the future.

Observation

When the researcher is concerned with habits and other attributes that may be difficult to elicit by the use of survey instruments, there are a number of observational techniques that lend themselves to description and analysis of behavior.

The structured checklist is one technique used for observation. What happens and how frequently it happens is recorded to determine the frequency of certain events or activities. For example, a study's purpose might be to determine if laryngectomy patients behave differently as a result of structured preoperative teaching about their surgery, as opposed to a different kind of instruction. The researcher creates a checklist of significant behaviors of the patients being observed in the study. The researcher then determines the frequencies of occurrence and tallies the results. This provides a foundation for interpretations and conclusions about the effect of structured preoperative teaching on the postoperative behavior of laryngectomy patients.

Observation research often requires that several observers be used. This means that there is a potential for differences of observations among the observers. Consequently, the researcher must be extremely careful to train observers by providing common experiences so that observer reliability can be established. Given the example of the laryngectomy patient study, observers could be shown films or videotapes of patients performing a range of behaviors. The observers would then mark the designated activities on their observation checklist, and their perceptions could be checked by the researcher. After a number of training sessions, interobserver reliability could be determined by correlational techniques.

Qualitative Strategies for Descriptive Research

Qualitative research studies are significantly more time consuming to conduct and analyze than quantitative research studies. Although qualitative research strategies appear deceptively simple on the surface, they require the researcher to spend enough time with the study subjects to obtain and analyze the data. The time required for collecting data can be very long, and data analysis can become very complex because of the many possible ways that the data can be analyzed and reduced to comprehensible information. The qualitative researcher must identify a researchable problem and design the study in the same fashion as the quantitative researcher, although testing hypotheses is neither required nor possible in many instances.

Phenomenology

Phenomenologic research is based on the philosophy of phenomenology, which was espoused by Edmund Husserl. Husserl's contention was that "meaning" is a personal experience that can be shared or communicated with others in an objective fashion and can be reduced to an underlying structure that can be understood by all individuals.

The phenomenologic researcher develops a research question that can be analyzed by the researcher based on the "feelings" of the research subjects concerning the phenomena being investigated. This can be done by asking the subjects to write their thoughts, feelings, and perceptions concerning the phenomena, as was done by Parse, Coyne, and Smith when they asked their subjects to describe, in writing, a time when they felt healthy [2]. The researchers then reviewed the subjects' writings for common themes, which they reduced to common "meanings."

The researcher may also be directly involved in the experience(s) being examined. In this case, the researcher observes and records the verbal and nonverbal actions of the subjects as well as their reaction(s) to the situation. Data may be collected through notes or other appropriate data-gathering techniques. Because any portion of the information may lead to the determination of "meanings," the researcher must be objective in recording the data.

Partial data analysis may take place during the data-collection phase. Since the researcher's goal is to reduce the myriad of observed phenomena to common elements, it may be possible to discover emergent themes very early on while collecting data. It must be noted, however, that the emergent themes or patterns may not contain substantive information and must be carefully scrutinized in light of the total data collected.

Researchers may use a judge panel of experts to determine whether the categories of meaning are valid [3]. Conversely, the researcher may opt to make the decisions concerning the categories of meaning and to establish their relative levels of importance.

Ethnography

Ethnographic research, often referred to as participant observation, may be used when the researcher must catalog all activities, or as many as possible, that are taking place in a social situation and then determine which activities are significant and which are trivial. This, essentially, is the technique used by social anthropologists or ethnographers. The social anthropologic researcher often becomes a participant as well as an observer and attempts to elicit data by using both structured and unstructured interviews and observations.

For example, there are many ways to examine beliefs about diseases and how to effect cures of these diseases. There are also many groups of people in developed as well as underdeveloped countries who practice various kinds of folk medicine to achieve cures. Disease etiology and classification are important to a nurse who is attempting to communicate with a patient. How the illness experience is perceived and described by a subculture is also a critical area for research. For example, the student who wrote the proposal in Appendix C proposed to describe what living in the congregate setting is like from the perspective of the homeless person with AIDS.

Other studies for which participant observation could be used include disease classification among Spanish-speaking migrant workers, the root medicine still practiced in many areas of the rural South, the continuation of various healing activities of Native-American groups, the introduction of herbal cures by different refugee groups, and the use of health foods and herbs in the population at large.

There are four levels of participant observation. The first level is that of a complete observer. If a researcher is working with a group of individuals whose language is not adequately understood or if discourse must be conducted through an interpreter, the researcher will be primarily an observer.

At the second level of participant observation, the researcher may become a partial participant. This could take place where the observer has a degree of fluency in the language and a great deal of knowledge concerning the group being studied. For example, a researcher working in a hospital setting might well fulfill this role. It is clear that the researcher is not a nurse, doctor, or member of the support staff of the hospital. This does not mean the researcher might not help in certain activities. Rather, it simply means that the researcher is nonjudgmental. Thus, the researcher can look for a variety of patterns of behaviors, social interactions, rituals, and other activities that are considered routine by the participants.

The third level of participant observation is that of an observer as participant. In this instance, a member of the group plays a dual role: first as a participating member of the group, with all of the rights and duties required of such a member, and second as an announced observer, where the group members are aware that they are being observed. As an example, a critical care nurse could describe the varieties of activities and interactions that occur between the various staff members in the critical care unit of a hospital. Some of the interactions would clearly be related to social and role expectations, rather than those interactions required to care for patients. Here the line between participant and observer is very narrow. Individuals within the group would know they were being observed, yet the observer would be able to perform the role of participant competently.

Finally, there is the role of full participant. The researcher conceals any intent to do research, and the subjects are not necessarily aware of the researcher's purpose. There are strong ethical questions involved in this type of research. Given the nature of informed consent by subjects in a research setting, total concealment of the research activity may be impossible.

It is the responsibility of the participant observer to make frequent and valid notes. Time considerations force many observers to develop a kind of shorthand for jotting down observations made on the spot. Later, the observers write down a full description of the event or events. Common sense dictates that such observations be recorded in full as soon as possible so that the researcher does not forget what those scribbles really meant.

The researcher who uses participant observation is limited as to the number of individuals with whom contacts can be made. The first contacts may be with marginal individuals who need social contacts and/or approval and whose information may be unreliable. Therefore, the researcher must be very careful that the data gathered are accurate and valid. A study of witchcraft beliefs might be extremely hard to document, for example, because of respondents' fear that they might be accused of witchcraft, or that they would become victims of witchcraft if they tell of known witches. Rapport and trust are crucial if the researcher is to obtain any kind of valid information.

Ethnographic researchers employ a technique called *key informant interviewing*. Key informants are those individuals whose positions or roles in a society or institution place them in a position to "know" what is really taking place. The participant observer must identify such individuals and gain their trust in order to have opportunities to interview them. Because key informants may be extremely busy individuals, care must be exercised not to waste their time and to take advantage of time that is unscheduled or at least free enough that the key informant does not feel that the investigator is too intrusive.

Grounded Theory

Grounded theory strategies were first reported by Glaser and Strauss when they examined the politics of pain management in a hospital environment [4]. Because there was little available existing data and no previously developed theory of pain management, the researchers had to collect data with no recourse to established ideas. This led to the strategy of the "constant comparative" method in which all the data being collected are compared to all the data previously collected in order to determine their importance and position in the hierarchy of data analysis. All kinds of data are collected. Written records and any other available data, such as verbal and nonverbal communications, are examined for their potential usefulness in the development of a usable theoretical framework. This means that the data collection and the data analysis stages of the research process occur simultaneously. The data are arranged in categories as patterns emerge. In the initial stages, the categories may be too broad or may be incorrect. As more data are collected, an isolated datum may be fitted into the appropriate category with greater ease.

After the researcher has developed categories, a framework is generated and a central hypothesis or theme may be formed concerning a key or core variable. The core variable is used to explain and simplify the complex structure of interactions that has been observed by the investigator(s).

Summary

In summary, the descriptive research approach is present-oriented in that it describes what now exists. In each case, the techniques and instruments must be carefully selected and evaluated to determine their appropriateness for collecting the study data. Careful attention must be paid to the fundamental questions of validity, reliability, and usability, as well as to time and cost constraints.

In order to apply the principles presented, you should complete the Workbook Activities.

References

1. Webb, Eugene, et al. 1966. *Unobtrusive Measures: Non-Reactive Research in the Social Sciences.* Chicago: Rand McNally, pp. 45–46.
2. Parse, R. R., A. B. Coyne, and M. J. Smith. 1985. *Nursing Research: Qualitative Methods.* Bowie, MD: Brady Communications.
3. Omery, A. 1983. "Phenomenology: A Method for Nursing Research." *Advances in Nursing Science,* 5: 49–63.
4. Glaser, B., and A. Strauss. 1967. *The Discovery of Grounded Theory: Strategies for Qualitative Research.* Chicago: Aldine.

Bibliography and Suggested Readings

Anastasi, A. 1976. *Psychological Testing,* 4th ed. New York: Macmillan.
Bromley, D. B. 1986. *The Case Study Method in Psychology and Related Research.* Chichester, NY: Wiley.

Dobbert, M. L. 1982. *Ethnographic Research.* New York: Praeger.

Glaser, B., and A. Strauss. 1967. *The Discovery of Grounded Theory: Strategies for Qualitative Research.* Chicago: Aldine.

Harrison, L. L. 1989. "Interfacing Bioinstruments with Computers for Data Collection." *Research in Nursing and Health,* 12 (February): 57–63.

Kalish, P. A., B. J. Kalish, and J. Clinton. 1982. "The World of Nursing on Prime Time Television, 1950 to 1980." *Nursing Research,* 31 (November–December): 358–363.

Lindeman, C. A. 1981. *Priorities within the Health Care System: A Delphi Study.* Kansas City: American Nurses' Association.

Linstone, H., and M. Turoo, Eds. 1975. *The Delphi Method: Techniques and Applications.* Reading, MA: Addison-Wesley.

Omery, A. 1983. "Phenomenology: A Method for Nursing Research." *Advances in Nursing Science,* 5: 49–63.

Osgood, C. E., G. J. Suci, and P. H. Tannenbaum. 1957. *The Structure of Inquiry.* Urbana: University of Illinois Press.

Parse, R. R., A. B. Coyne, and M. J. Smith. 1985. *Nursing Research: Qualitative Methods.* Bowie, MA: Brady Communications.

Poyatos, F., Ed. 1988. *Cross Cultural Perspectives in Nonverbal Communication.* Toronto: Hogrefe.

Rosengren, K. E., Ed. 1981. *Advances in Content Analysis.* Beverly Hills, CA: Sage.

Rosenthal, R. 1966. *Experimenter Effects in Behavioral Research.* New York: Appleton-Century-Crofts.

Sackman, H. 1975. *Delphi Critique: Expert Opinion, Forecasting, and Group Process.* Lexington, MA: Lexington Books.

Turner, A. P. F., I. Karube, and G. Wilson. 1987. *Biosensors: Fundamentals and Applications.* Oxford: Oxford University Press.

Webb, E., et al., 1981. *Nonreactive Measures in the Social Sciences.* Boston: Houghton Mifflin.

Webb, E., D. T. Campbell, R. D. Schwartz, and L. Sechrest. 1966. *Unobtrusive Measures: Nonreactive Research in the Social Sciences.* Chicago: Rand McNally.

Weiman, J. M., and R. D. Harrison, Eds. 1983. *Nonverbal Interaction.* Beverly Hills, CA: Sage.

Werner, O., and G. M. Schoepfle. 1987. *Systematic Fieldwork.* Beverly Hills, CA: Sage.

Yin, R. K. 1984. *Case Study Research.* Beverly Hills, CA: Sage.

9 The Experimental Research Approach

Objectives

When you have finished reading this chapter you should be able to:

1. Compare common experimental research designs

2. Identify strengths and weaknesses of experimental research designs

3. Describe why the results of an ex post facto study may be called into question

4. Identify effects that may have negative impact on a research study

5. Discuss the difference between quasi-experimental and true experimental research designs

6. Describe the advantages of blind studies in experimental research

---

The Nature of Experimental Research
Quasi-Experimental Research Designs
Experimental Research Designs
    One-Group Pretest–Posttest Design
    Pretest–Posttest Control Group
    Matching Samples
    Solomon Four-Group Design
    Two-Group Random Sample
    Nonrandomized Control Group Design
    Counterbalanced Design
    Time Series Design
    Control Group Time Series Design
    Factorial Designs
    Ex Post Facto Designs—Correlations
Considerations in Experimental Research Design
    Generalizability
    Subject Sensitization
    Replicability
    Historical Factors
    Fatigue

The material in this chapter is designed to introduce you to some basic principles and methods of the experimental design approach. When researching a nursing problem, we seek solutions that we hope will improve patient care and enhance the quality of life for all people. One of the greatest problems we face in seeking solutions to research problems is that we are dealing with human subjects, who may report a wide variety of feelings, attitudes, or even misunderstandings. Obviously, the researcher wants to control as many factors as possible. This leads to the use of an experimental approach and the development of experimental design methodology.

The Nature of Experimental Research

Experimental design is based on the notion of control. Observed instances of an activity may or may not be the cause of an observed consequence. The experimenter wants to determine if the activity was or was not the cause of the effect observed. For example, parents, teachers, and others admonish children not to get their feet wet because the children will catch cold. Although this may seem to be a reasonable admonition, in fact, we know that colds are caused by viruses that are transmitted from one person to another. Wet feet in and of themselves will not cause a person to catch a cold. They may make the person uncomfortable, disturb physiologic balance, and lower resistance to infection; but, alone, foot wetting is not the causal factor in colds. Many common-sense ideas are rooted in the folklore of cause and effect; the careful researcher designs experiments to verify if, indeed, the cause does bring about the observed effect.

As has been mentioned, working with human subjects makes experimental research extremely difficult. Controls are difficult to apply, and many techniques used on plants and animals are certainly not open to experimenters who work with human subjects. Reexamine the discussion of the protection of human subjects in Chapter 4 to gain a fuller appreciation of the researcher's responsibilities for the protection of human rights.

It is again worthwhile to mention the idea of statistical significance. A desired level of outcome is established prior to carrying out the research plan. Frequently, the result is not statistically significant, and the researcher goes away feeling that the research was for naught. Nothing could be further from the truth. Research studies that yield no statistical significance, if carefully planned and executed, are just as valid as studies that yield statistically significant differences. Beginning researchers sometimes have the idea that their research is not acceptable if no statistically significant difference is found. Most researchers want to reject the null hypothesis. They believe the experimental approach they are using is better than some other approach, and they often have a vested interest in the success of their experiments. They find it terribly disappointing to discover that their great ideas did not work out as expected.

In reviewing the literature, we quickly discover that research journals tend to report studies with highly significant results. This attitude has developed over the years and is potentially damaging to the research process. Editors of some journals will report only those reports that are highly significant but will not report equally valid studies that show no statistically significant differences.

Organizations that give grant funds often like to have significant results. A researcher whose experiments show no significant difference may be less likely to be funded a second time than a researcher whose experiments show such differences. Unfortunately, this has led to a number of false reports by unethical researchers.

We must remember that the field of statistics developed outside of the area of human subject research. Experimental rigor can be applied far more effectively by experimenters who work with biological or physical specimens, and who can more easily control the variables to analyze their experimental results, than by those who work with human subjects.

Finally, even a slight improvement in a condition may be significant to the individuals with that condition, even though the treatment may not be statistically significant as far as the controlled experiment is concerned.

Up to now we have referred frequently to the word *control,* which can be defined as a manipulation or alteration of the experimental conditions in order to limit sources of error. As described in Chapter 6, the purpose of experimental research is to determine if condition X (the cause) will result in response Y (the effect). Condition X is termed the *independent variable,* and response Y is the *dependent variable.*

The nature of control is to restrict the effects of *extraneous variables* that could have an impact on the variables under investigation and could affect the outcome of the research.

Careful controls are also used to avoid side effects that could occur during the course of a potentially harmful experiment. Many useful drugs may be highly toxic or have unpleasant side effects if doses are too large. For example, reports of experiments with rats and mice by the Food and Drug Administration caused a great furor by identifying artificial sweeteners, such as cyclamates and saccharin, as potential carcinogens. These experiments were conducted in such a manner that the quantities of potentially harmful substances to be ingested by the experimental animals were carefully controlled. By varying the quantity levels of the substances, the experimenters could determine differential responses to the substances. Also, the Surgeon General's reports are able to state with higher and higher degrees of certainty that the more one smokes, the greater one's odds of having various medical problems.

Probably the most important control the experimenter uses is that of random assignments of subjects to groups (also called *randomization*). Every subject should have an equal chance of being assigned to any group as the investigator assigns subjects to a control group or an experimental group on a random basis. The purpose of random assignment is to avoid any systematic bias in the groups being studied.

Quasi-Experimental Research Designs

Sometimes the researcher is not able to design a true experimental study because of constraints imposed in subject selection or the setting of the study. In such cases, the researcher may use a quasi-experimental design, in which the investigator can manipulate the independent variable (the experimental condition) and exercise some control over the experiment. However, random assignment of subjects to control or experimental groups is not feasible. For example, a researcher may want to investigate the differences between patients who may or may not receive a certain protocol, as routinely ordered by different physicians. That is, physician A might never order the protocol, physician B always orders the protocol at a set time, and physician C always orders the protocol at a set time different from physician B's time. In this case, the researcher cannot randomly assign the study subjects to the treatment groups even though the impact of the time of the protocol or the lack of it can be measured. This is in contrast to the true experimental design of a study in which a researcher would be able to randomly assign the study subjects to either the experimental or the control group.

Experimental Research Designs

There are a number of ways to design true experimental research. Each design is characterized by manipulation of the independent variable by the investigator, and by some form of control and randomization. The designs range from simple to extremely complex.

One-Group Pretest–Posttest Design

The simplest type of experimental design is the *one-group pretest–posttest design*. Although this design leaves many things to chance, it is often the only available way to determine the effectiveness of a treatment. Essentially, this design measures what has happened to the experimental group based on the way it was prior to the beginning of the experiment (pretest state), and the differences achieved at the end of the experiment (posttest state).

For example, such a design might be used to study a group of patients who suffer mild angina pain. The experimenter could measure cholesterol level in the patients' blood and then ask the patients to restrict their intake of cholesterol through changes in their diets. After a given period of time, the experimenter would determine whether or not the mild angina pain had been reduced and if the blood cholesterol levels had dropped. If blood cholesterol levels had dropped and angina pain has been reduced, the experimenter might then conclude that lowering cholesterol levels in the blood reduces angina pain. Note that there is a minimal amount of control placed on other variables that might affect the evidence in the study subjects. Changes in stress patterns, weight, exercise patterns, or any one of many other factors might have contributed to the change.

The following example shows the characteristics of the one-group pretest–posttest design:

Number of Groups Used	Pretest?	Treatment?	Posttest?	Strength of Design
1	Yes	Yes	Yes	Weak

Pretest–Posttest Control Group

A second and more sophisticated technique of experimentation is the use of a *control group* to determine if the treatment appears to make a difference. Utilizing the previous cholesterol example, a number of subjects with mild angina pain would be randomly assigned to two groups: an *experimental group* and a *control group*. The experimental group subjects would then alter their diets, while the control group subjects would change nothing. At the end of the experiment, the researcher would determine whether there was a significant difference in the cholesterol levels of both groups. If this difference was significant, and there was a significant difference in the reported incidences of mild angina pain between the experimental and the control group, the experimenter could then conclude that the reduction of blood cholesterol did have an effect on the occurrence of angina.

Note that there was no attempt to match or otherwise compare the members of either group. The only common element of control the control group shares with the experimental group is mild angina pain. Note also the term *mild*. Pain perception varies greatly from individual to individual, and response to pain varies between cultures as well as between the sexes within a culture. In the previous example, not all of these factors were taken into consideration, only the common diagnosis of mild angina pain.

The following example shows the characteristics of the pretest–posttest control group design: X refers to the experimental group; C refers to the control group.

Number of Groups Used	Pretest?	Treatment?	Posttest?	Strength of Design
2	X Yes C Yes	X Yes C No	X Yes C Yes	Weak

Matching Samples

Far more valuable in terms of rigor would be a research design that attempts to match or to pair the control and the experimental group. In the cholesterol study, the experimenter might use simple matching procedures such as height, weight, sex, age, and smoking or nonsmoking, or such sophisticated measurements as psychological stress tests, projective techniques, or any one of literally dozens of methods in order to control for extraneous variables.

A major problem with this type of experimental design is that, unless the subject pool is infinitely large, the experimenter reduces the available sample with each matching or pairing situation. Males can be matched only with other males. Age further reduces the sample size. Eventually, it is entirely possible to reduce the sample down to two very well matched individuals. The problem then becomes one of a large enough sample size to be generalizable to the target population.

The following example shows the characteristics of the matching sample design: X refers to the experimental group; C refers to the control group.

Number of Groups Used	Pretest?	Treatment?	Posttest?	Strength of Design
2	X Yes C Yes	X Yes C No	X Yes C Yes	Weak

Solomon Four-Group Design

A frequently used and highly valid experimental procedure is the *Solomon four-group design*. An experimenter using this methodology randomly divides the sample into four separate groups. Effectively, there are two experimental groups and two control groups.

The first experimental group receives the same procedures as in the pretest–posttest design. Subjects are randomly selected, pretested, given the appropriate treatment, and then given the posttest.

The first of the control groups is given the pretest, no treatment, and then the posttest. Up to this point, the Solomon design is precisely the same as the pretest–posttest control group design. However, group 3 is also defined as an experimental group. In our cholesterol example, it would consist of subjects diagnosed as having mild angina. They would not be given the pretest; that is, their cholesterol level would not be measured at all. However, they would receive the treatment; that is, their intake of cholesterol would be reduced and they would be given the appropriate blood tests at the end of the experimental period.

Subjects in the fourth group in the Solomon design would have nothing done until the posttest. They would not be pretested for cholesterol levels at the experiment's beginning and they would not receive any treatment. Only at the end of the experiment would their blood cholesterol level be measured (posttested) and then compared to the incidence of anginal pain in the other groups.

Because two of the groups (groups 1 and 3) have received the experimental treatment, any differences noted by the experimenter can be more confidently ascribed to the treatment if both experimental groups show similar results at the end of the treatment and there is a significant difference between the experimental and the control groups. Similarly, a lack of significant difference between the four groups enables the investigator to accept the null hypothesis.

The following example shows the characteristics of the Solomon four-group design: X refers to the experimental group; C refers to the control group.

Number of Groups Used	Pretest?	Treatment?	Posttest?	Strength of Design
4	X1 Yes	X1 Yes	X1 Yes	Strong
	C1 Yes	C1 No	C1 Yes	
	X2 No	X2 Yes	X2 Yes	
	C2 No	C2 No	C2 Yes	

Two-Group Random Sample

The experimenter may choose to use only the last two groups of the Solomon design. That is, one group is given the treatment and then posttested with no pretesting, and the control group is given only the posttest. The theory behind this methodology is that the experimenter, adhering rigorously to the random assignment of subjects to the groups, can say that the two groups were essentially the same because random assignment should avoid any systematic bias in the two groups.

This type of design simplifies the experimenter's task and eliminates the effect of a pretest on the subjects. In effect, it maintains the subjects' naiveté. It is also noteworthy that there are some things that cannot be pretested or accurately predicted. Patients who are already suffering from mild angina pain may or may not be suffering from elevated cholesterol levels. The angina pain already exists. If treatment or lack of treatment (cholesterol in the diet) is a factor, there should be a difference between the two groups at the end of the treatment.

The following example shows the characteristics of the two-group random sample design: X refers to the experimental group; C refers to the control group.

Number of Groups Used	Pretest?	Treatment?	Posttest?	Strength of Design
2	X No	X Yes	X Yes	Strong
	C No	C No	C Yes	

Nonrandomized Control Group Design

Occasionally, circumstances may preclude random assignment of subjects to groups at the beginning of an experiment. For example, the experimenter may wish to compare a sample of individuals from a local Veteran's Administration hospital with a sample of individuals from a privately funded hospital who are also complaining of angina pain. One of the hospitals may insist on a standardized routine of treatment for angina patients, whereas the other hospital may be available for the experimental treatment.

In this case, the subjects in both samples are given the pretest and one group is given the experimental treatment, but the researcher is not able to control various interaction effects at the beginning of the experiment. In this instance, where it is not possible to develop controls by assigning subjects randomly to control and experimental groups, alternative methods of statistical analysis are required. The method commonly used is the analysis of covariance; a statistical technique that allows the experimenter to control for varying potential interaction effects after the experiment has been performed.

The following example shows the characteristics of the nonrandomized control group design: X refers to the experimental group; C refers to the control group.

Number of Groups Used	Pretest?	Treatment?	Posttest?	Strength of Design
2	X Yes C Yes	X Yes C No	X Yes C Yes	Control through analysis of covariance can be strong

Counterbalanced Design

A more effective design, or at least one that attempts to remove some of the previously described problems, is the *counterbalanced design*. This design can be used when more than one treatment method is attempted. Each set of subjects is given the treatment at the same point in time during the course of the experiment. This means that sets of subjects become both experimental and control groups for themselves and for another group. Because of the nonrandom nature of group assignments, the experimenter cannot control differences. However, the testing does allow for greater flexibility in the interpretation of results; differences are noted both between groups and within groups. Utilizing the statistical test of analysis of variance, the experimenter may be able to determine that the effects were caused by the treatment.

For example, a group of psychiatric patients might be subjected to a computer program designed to interact with individuals and give the illusion of eliciting feelings. (Such a program exists and may be found on many college campuses as either "Doctor" or "Eliza.") After such interaction, the subjects would then be given a subjective test and their responses scored. At an alternative time, standard psychotherapeutic techniques would be used and the same projective tests would be given. After a number of alternating treatments, types of responses to the projective tests could be measured, and the differences, if any, between the two treatments could be recorded.

A number of variations to this design should be noted. Two or more variables could be introduced, such as another type of treatment in addition to computer and psychotherapy. Perhaps a questionnaire could be utilized with a format such as "I feel _____." Here the subject chooses from a list of adjectives provided and is then asked to tell why he or she feels this way. Or a question such as "How do you feel about _____?" could be asked. Responses to projective techniques could again be used to determine differences between the treatments.

The following example shows the characteristics of the counterbalanced design: X refers to the experimental group; C refers to the control group.

Number of Groups Used	Pretest?	Treatment?	Posttest?	Strength of Design
		Treatment A		
Varies (X's and C's reverse roles in study)	X Yes C Yes	X Yes C No	X Yes C Yes	Strong
		Treatment B		
	X Yes C Yes	X No C Yes	X Yes C Yes	

Time Series Design

Most experimental studies fall into two categories: one-shot studies and those that continue over a longer period of time, known as longitudinal studies. As an experimenter you may want to measure the effects of a treatment over a long period of time. You would thus continue to administer the treatment and would measure the effects a number of times during the course of the experiment.

In our cholesterol example, instead of testing patients with mild angina pain only once (at the end of the diet restriction), the design would call for testing at stated intervals. Chemical or behavioral changes in a human being can be very subtle and difficult to measure. Responses can vary daily, and some intervening but unrecognized variables may lead to incorrect conclusions. Testing over a long period of time helps to reduce such pitfalls and improves the experiment. With a time series experiment, however, variables occurring during and after treatment may go unnoticed by the experimenter and can lead to a false or improper conclusion.

The following example shows the characteristics of the time series design: X refers to the experimental group; C refers to the control group.

Number of Groups Used	Pretest?	Treatment?	Posttest?	Strength of Design
1	Yes	Yes over time	Yes over time	Strong

Control Group Time Series Design

In order to diminish the problems inherent in a time series design, experimenters can use a *control group time series design*. This design requires that a control group be tested simultaneously with the experimental group without being given the treatment. In our cholesterol example, two groups of randomly selected angina patients would receive a sequential series of blood tests over a period of time. The experimenter would then determine if blood cholesterol had diminished significantly between the experimental treatment group and the control group, as well as the frequency and intensity of angina pain. This technique, obviously, provides far greater control than a single time series design and is preferable to the single time series design.

The following example shows the characteristics of the control group time series design: X refers to the experimental group; C refers to the control group.

Number of Groups Used	Pretest?	Treatment?	Posttest?	Strength of Design
2	X Yes	X Yes over time	X Yes over time	Strong
	C Yes	C No over time	C Yes over time	

Factorial Designs

In experimental designs like those we have been discussing, the experimenter identifies one independent variable and one dependent variable. Through the use of various forms of control, the effect of the independent variable on the dependent variable is then measured. However, there may be a time when we find that there are two or more variables that occurred simultaneously and, through interaction, may cause the dependent variable to appear in the way that it did.

Using our cholesterol example, suppose the subjects were overweight when placed on the low-cholesterol diet. In some cases weight might be maintained because, although saturated fat intake is reduced, there is a plethora of nonsaturated fats that could be substituted for the saturated fats.

The experimenter, however, might want to reduce both the weight and the intake of saturated fats of the subjects simultaneously. At the end of the experiment, it might be found that angina pain had been reduced in both intensity and frequency. It would then become very difficult to ascribe the causal effects to either of the two independent variables. Experimenters can more easily control experiments in which one and only one independent variable is introduced, as in the case of a cholesterol intake reduction alone or a weight-loss diet alone. Often the interaction of two or more variables produces more significant results than a single variable does. The experimenter must then use what is called a *factorial design*. In this type of design, subjects are divided into all possible combinations to determine the effect of the independent variables alone and the effect of the interaction of the independent variables.

Such factorial designs can grow to enormous complexity very quickly, but such is the work of researchers. Human beings are enormously complex; even the simplest, most tightly designed and tightly controlled experiment has results that are probably influenced by interaction effects. Factorial designs attempt to get at these interactive effects and determine their impact on the experiment.

The following example shows the characteristics of the factorial design: X refers to the experimental group; C refers to the control group.

Number of Groups Used	Pretest?	Treatment?	Posttest?	Strength of Design
Varies	X Yes C Varies	X Yes C Varies	X Yes C Yes	Strong but can be very complex

Table 9-1 summarizes the experimental designs using the diagrammatic explanation of each design.

Ex Post Facto Designs—Correlations

In *ex post facto research,* changes in the independent variable have already occurred prior to the research. Ex post facto designs are really correlational designs that allow the researcher to infer relationships among variables, rather than draw cause-and-effect conclusions. This can lead to spurious (incorrect) conclusions. Researchers who conclude that a high positive or high negative correlation is necessarily a cause-and-effect relationship have failed to see the whole picture. There is a tendency to oversimplify in drawing conclusions. It has been said that there are two solutions to every problem: one short, simple, and wrong and the other extremely complicated. Indeed, there has been a problem regarding the reports of several regulatory agencies of the federal government, such as the Food and Drug Administration and the Surgeon General's office, both of which have reported a great deal of correlational research. Because of the potential ambiguity in interpretation, industries such as the tobacco industry and the artificial sweetener industry have often attempted—and sometimes succeeded—in responding to these reports with other correlational studies of their own showing lower relationships or no causality at all. This has led to much confusion on the consumer's part because the question of whom to believe looms large when dealing with such complex market issues.

In summary, true experimental research design is characterized by ma-

Table 9-1. Comparison of Experimental Designs

Design	Number of Groups Used	Pretest?	Treatment?	Posttest?	Strength of Design
One-group pretest/post-test	1	Yes	Yes	Yes	Weak
Pretest/postest control group	2	X[a] Yes C[b] Yes	X Yes C No	X Yes C Yes	Weak
Matching samples	2	X Yes C Yes	X Yes C No	X Yes C Yes	Weak
Solomon four-group design	4	X1 Yes C1 Yes X2 No C2 No	X1 Yes C1 No X2 Yes C2 No	X1 Yes C1 Yes X2 Yes C2 Yes	Strong
Two-group random sample	2	X No C No	X Yes C No	X Yes C Yes	Strong
Nonrandomized control group	2	X Yes C Yes	X Yes C No	X Yes C Yes	Control through analysis of covariance can be strong
Counterbalanced	Varies (X's and C's reverse roles in study)	*Treatment A* X Yes C Yes *Treatment B* X Yes C Yes	*Treatment A* X Yes C No *Treatment B* X No C Yes	*Treatment A* X Yes C Yes *Treatment B* X Yes C Yes	Strong
Time series	1	Yes	Yes over time	Yes over time	Strong
Control group time series	2	X Yes C Yes	X Yes over time C No over time	X Yes over time C Yes over time	Strong
Factorial	Varies	X Yes C Varies	X Yes C Varies	X Yes C Yes	Strong but can be very complex

[a]X refers to experimental group(s).
[b]C refers to control group(s).

nipulation of the independent variable by the investigator, who exercises some form of control over the experimental situation, including random assignment of subjects to groups (randomization).

Considerations in Experimental Research Design

In all true experimental studies, the researcher must keep several concerns as high-priority items when designing research.

Generalizability

The researcher should design the experiment so that its findings will be generalizable to the larger target population when sampling techniques are used. Sometimes research studies do not allow for generalization because of sample size, method of subject selection, or various other reasons. In addition, experiments carried out in artificial or restricted laboratory situations often preclude generalizability. Quasi-experimental designs are less generalizable than true experimental designs.

Subject Sensitization

Subjects can become sensitized or knowledgeable about the procedures used. This is especially true where a psychological rather than a physiologic response is measured. By its very nature, a pretest gives information about what it is the experimenter wants to discover. Even if questions are masked, subjects will know something about the research. Even physiologic measurements can be affected. With our increased knowledge of biofeedback, we can see that subjects may be able to control, voluntarily or involuntarily, many of their physiologic responses.

Replicability

Can the research be repeated in another setting with other subjects? If a study can be replicated, and other researchers get similar results, a great deal more confidence can be placed in the conclusions drawn by the original researchers. One of the criteria for developing a scientific research base for utilization in nursing practice is sufficient replication of the studies to ensure the validity of the results of the studies.

Historical Factors

Historical factors may also come into play. If an experiment is carried out over a period of time, events extraneous to the experiment, such as maturation or increased knowledge on the part of the subjects, may cause changes. These events become intervening variables and must be accounted for.

Fatigue

Both the subjects and the researchers can become fatigued, bored, or inattentive during the course of a research study. This means treatment, or response measurement, may not be consistent during the course of an experiment. There comes a time when both subjects and researchers have the feeling of "let's get this thing over with and get out of here." This natural fatigue must be guarded against in order to ensure correct and consistent measurement.

Attrition

In research conducted over a period of time, there may be attrition or loss of subjects. Subjects move, become ill, withdraw because they are tired of the research, or are lost to the experiment for any number of other reasons. This means that an experimenter who starts with too small a sample or samples at the beginning of the experiment may obtain insufficient data for valid analysis.

Hawthorne Effect

Over the years there have been many studies of the Hawthorne effect. The Hawthorne studies were a series of classic studies conducted in the late 1920s and early 1930s at the Hawthorne Plant of the Western Electric Company in Chicago. The *Hawthorne effect* is the term used to describe the psychological reactions to the presence of the investigator or to special treatment during the study, which tends to alter the responses of the subjects. Subjects may change their behavior in an effort to please the experimenter. Again, we caution that experimenters can unconsciously bias subjects merely by their tone of voice or facial expression.

Experimenter Bias

Sometimes experimenter expectations interfere with the gathering of accurate results. Many experimenters have a vested interest in their experiments, and failure to reject the null hypothesis may be a terrible blow to one's ego. A true researcher remains objective and attempts to control as many variables as possible.

Blind Studies

Methods called *blind studies* have been developed to ensure that experimenter bias and the Hawthorne effect are reduced or eliminated. *Single blind* studies may be carried out in one of two ways. In one method of single blind studies, the subjects know whether they are in the experimental group or the control group, but the experimenter does not know which group each subject is in. In the other single blind method, the experimenter knows which group the subjects are in, but the subjects do not know which group they are in. The preferred method of blind studies is the *double blind* study, where only an outside, neutral party has assigned subjects to the experimental and control groups, and neither subjects nor experimenter knows which subjects are in which group.

Summary

In summary, we have discussed the nature of experimental research and a number of the most commonly used experimental research designs, including the one-group pretest–posttest design; the pretest–posttest control group design; the matching sample design; the Solomon four-group design; the two-group random sample design; the nonrandomized control group design; the counterbalanced design; the time series design; the control group time series design; factorial designs; and ex post facto designs. We have also discussed the nature of quasi-experimental research as well as some considerations in experimental research design. Beginning researchers should be aware that there are other less common designs that may be found in the literature.

In order to apply the principles presented, you should complete the Workbook Activities at the end of this text.

Bibliography and Suggested Readings

Broota, K. D. 1989. *Experimental Design in Behavioral Research.* New York: Wiley.

Campbell, D. T., and J. Stanley. 1963. *Experimental and Quasi-Experimental Designs for Research.* Chicago: Rand McNally.

Forcese, D. P., and S. Richer. 1973. *Social Research Methods.* Englewood Cliffs, NJ: Prentice-Hall.

Kerlinger, F. H. 1973. *Foundations of Behavioral Research,* 2nd ed. New York: Holt, Rinehart and Winston.

Kidder, L. H., C. M. Judd, and E. R. Smith. 1986. *Research Methods in Social Relations,* 5th ed. New York: Holt, Rinehart and Winston.

Polit, D., and B. Hungler. 1995. *Nursing Research: Principles and Methods,* 5th ed. Philadelphia: J. B. Lippincott.

Solomon, R. C. 1949. "An Extension of Control Group Design." *Psychological Bulletin,* 46: 137–150.

10 Data Analysis

Objectives

When you have finished reading this chapter you should be able to:

1. Define the following terms: Mean, Median, Mode, Standard Deviation

2. Describe four levels of measurement

3. Distinguish between descriptive and inferential statistics

4. Distinguish between parametric and nonparametric statistics

5. Describe the function of correlations

6. Understand the purpose of meta-analysis

> **Qualitative Data Analysis**
>   Phenomenology
>   Grounded Theory
>   Ethnography
> **The Use of Computers in Qualitative Data Analysis**

The purpose of this chapter is to acquaint you with some basic information about the analysis and interpretation of data in research studies. It should help you understand and evaluate different methods of treating both quantitative and qualitative data.

Quantitative Data Analysis

It is highly significant that statistical analysis in nursing research traces its roots back to Florence Nightingale. Although Nightingale lacked the sophisticated techniques available to the nurse researcher today, she did utilize and publish descriptive statistical analyses using graphs and charts concerning the mortality of soldiers during the Crimean War. For a brief review of Nightingale's statistical techniques, you might want to read Cohen's article in the March 1984 issue of *Scientific American* [1].

The Use of Statistics in Data Analysis

Statistics are ways of measuring things or groups of things. Any time we measure opinions, average numbers of miles per gallon, or the odds in a card game, we are using statistics. Basically, there are two kinds of statistics: descriptive and inferential. *Descriptive statistics* simply describe the population with which we are concerned. *Inferential statistics* allow us to draw other kinds of conclusions about a population based on a sample or samples, and to predict future happenings. Both quantitative and qualitative researchers may use a variety of statistical techniques to analyze their data. Quantitative researchers usually tend to use more complex statistical analyses than qualitative researchers.

Descriptive Statistics

Essentially, descriptive statistics describe. This type of statistical analysis is the simple reporting of facts and collective occurrences based on a number of samples. Sometimes the easiest way to describe a set of data is to draw a picture or pictures of the information. For example, suppose we had the following set of scores on a test.

7, 6, 8, 9, 10, 9, 7, 11, 11, 9, 9, 9, 10, 8, 8

It is very hard to make any sense out of such data. But if the researcher organized the data by making a histogram (graph), the results are much clearer (Fig. 10-1).

Another way to organize these data would be to make a bar graph (Fig. 10-2). This type of representation clearly shows the number of scores at each level of scoring.

A third way to show these data would be by the use of a frequency polygon. In this instance, the midpoints on the bar graph are connected and the bars are eliminated, so that the scores are as shown in Figure 10-3.

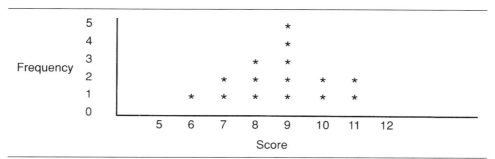

Fig. 10-1. Histogram

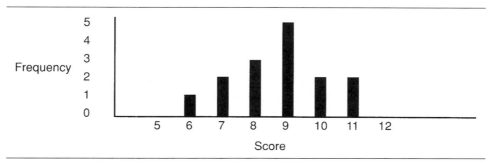

Fig. 10-2. Bar graph

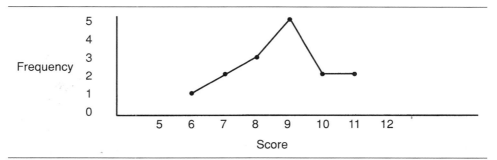

Fig. 10-3. Frequency polygon

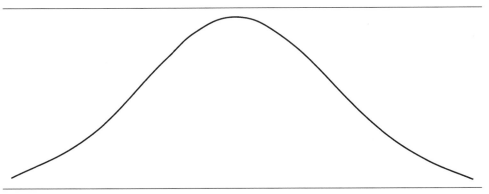

Fig. 10-4. Normal curve

As we can see, the corners of a frequency polygon can be smoothed out so that we get a figure resembling a normal curve (Fig. 10-4).

When we use descriptive statistics, we are concerned with several types of measures: (1) centrality or central tendency, (2) dispersion, and (3) location or position within the sample or the population.

If you were to measure any large population, you would find that the members of the population would distribute themselves across what is known as the *normal curve.*

The Mean

As you can see, most of the population clusters about the high point or the center of the curve. If the curve is perfectly symmetrical, the center of the normal curve is called the *mean.* Statistically, the mean is shown by the symbol $\bar{X}$. The mean may be thought of as the average. For example, suppose we have seven scores on a simple test:

$$5, 4, 3, 2, 6, 7, 8$$

When we add these scores and then divide the sum by the total number of tests, we find that 5 is the mean, or average, in this case.

Of course, means often describe essentially mythical characteristics. No one owns 1.3 cars or 2.2 television sets, or has 2.5 children. The mean gives us some idea of what a total population may be like, but it is not a measure in which we can put our complete trust. For example, suppose we have seven more scores from a test:

$$6, 7, 8, 5, 4, 10, 23$$

The mean of these seven scores is now 9. Yet only two scores are above 9.

Thus, this average implies something that does not accurately reflect what happened with the test scores. The curve is distorted.

The Median

When we have extreme scores that cause distortion of the curve, we can use another measure to show how central the mean really is. This is called the *median*. The median is the number that divides the sample in half, so that 50 percent of the sample falls above the median and 50 percent falls below. In our first example of seven scores, we find that the median is 5, the same as the mean. In the second example, however, the mean is 9, but the median is 7. In this particular instance, 7 is probably more descriptive of what is really happening.

The Mode

Still another measure of central tendency is the *mode*. This statistic tells us where scores tend to cluster. For example, consider these numbers:

4, 5, 6, 6, 6, 7, 8

The most frequently occurring score or number is 6. Consequently, the mode is 6. In this example the mean and the median also happen to be 6.

Remember, it is fairly unusual and inadvisable to use descriptive statistics exclusively with small samples. Using such techniques distorts the data analysis.

Percentile Rank

Measures that reflect the relative position of a score in a distribution are also descriptive in nature. One the most commonly used statistics is the *percentile rank*. The percentile rank is the point below which a percentage of scores occurs. In percentile rank, the median is always the fiftieth percentile. A person scoring at the sixtieth percentile is above 60 percent of the other test takers and below the other 40 percent.

Other percentage-based statistics commonly found in the literature are the decile (10 percent) and the quartile (25 percent). Means, medians, and modes are used when we want to describe central tendency. They give us an idea of how alike members of a population are. Sometimes, however, we want to know how a population is actually distributed over the curve. Then we must use measures of dispersion. The most frequently used measure of dispersion is the standard deviation.

The Standard Deviation

On all normal curves, certain proportions of the sample cluster around the mean. We can find out how widely distributed the scores are by measuring the *standard deviation*. When a curve is normal, about 68 percent of the population will be within one standard deviation, plus or minus, of the mean. We discuss the "average" characteristics of a population when we report the mean, but we usually consider this 68 percent (34 percent above the mean and 34 percent below the mean) to be within the normal or average range. Ninety-five percent of the population will be within two standard deviations from the mean, and 99.7 percent will be within three standard deviations (Fig. 10-5).

The important idea is not the percentages of the population that are contained under any portion of a curve but, rather, the shape of the curve. There is one standard (imaginary) bell-shaped curve that we have been using to illustrate the statistical curve. Curves can take many shapes, some with a narrow range and others with a wide range between standard deviations (Fig. 10-6).

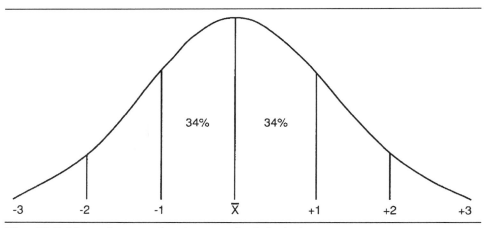

Fig. 10-5. Normal curve showing standard deviation

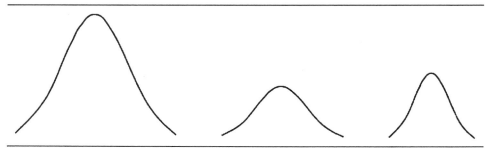

Fig. 10-6. Three normal curves

If a test is given and the standard deviation is found to be 2 and the mean 16, this means that 68 percent of the population will fall between the scores of 14 and 18 on the normal curve. If the standard deviation of the same test is 4, the curve will assume a different shape; if the standard deviation is 8, still another shape will be assumed. Consequently, we can always describe the shape of the curve on the basis of the standard deviation. We can also get some idea of the range of scores and a better feeling for an average individual.

Inferential Statistics

Descriptive statistics give us a quantitative way of viewing the world. They enable us to describe certain factual aspects of a population. Most researchers, however, are concerned with other kinds of judgments as well. This leads us to the use of *inferential statistics.* Inferential statistics do not examine a whole population. Rather, as described in Chapter 6, a sample or samples are drawn from the population and the characteristics of the population are deduced or inferred from the responses of this sample.

In addition to this type of *inference,* the researcher uses inferential statistics to determine whether certain experimental treatments or techniques are better, worse, or not significantly different from other types of treatments or techniques. This is called *hypothesis testing* and is based on probability. When reading research, the beginning researcher continually runs across the proposition $H = p < .05$. (Remember that H_0 is called the null hypothesis, as discussed in Chap. 5.) Here, $p < .05$ is called the *level of significance.* That is, the researcher states that the results will probably *not* be significantly different from the standard or common treatment. Most researchers really want to reject the null hypothesis, but research convention has cast this as the most common type of research hypothesis. The symbol p stands for probability. The probability in the statement $p < .05$ means that there will be no conclusion of a significant difference between treatments unless 5 or fewer treatments out of 100 have the same result as the original or standard treatment.

When a level of significance is selected, the experimenter is telling the world that chance has little to do with the results of the experiment. Medically related experiments may set extremely high levels of significance; usually, one chance in a thousand or less ($p < .001$). In cases of life and death, the chance of error must be diminished as much as possible.

Levels of Measurement

When dealing with inferential statistics, we must be concerned with what are called *levels of measurement.* Often, the researcher works with data represented by responses to questions that can be posed in various ways.

The Nominal Scale

The first level of data measurement is called the *nominal* level or nominal scale. The responses to this scale deal only with mutually exclusive data. There are no qualifiers. For example, we can classify all people in the world as having either blue eyes or brown eyes. If we choose to do this, anyone whose eyes are considered green, grey, or black must be placed in the category blue or brown. Nominal scales deal only with exclusive categories and do not attempt to find gradations between them. The categories are absolute, and the mode is the only measure of central tendency.

In nursing research, the nominal scale might be used to determine if pregnancies and abortions occur statistically more frequently in one of two socially different groups of women. This can be done by simply identifying members of one group or the other and asking each subject if she has ever had an abortion. The responses of each group could then be tallied and analyzed statistically to determine if there was a significant difference in the frequency of abortion between the two groups (Fig. 10-7).

The Ordinal Scale

The next highest level of measurement is called *ordinal* measurement. Subjects are asked to rank ideas, items, or other things. The subject can respond that item A is more or less than items B or C, but cannot tell exactly how much more or less. For example, a patient may experience more or less discomfort, depending on certain postures or other physical phenomena that can be adjusted. The amount cannot be quantified by saying, "I am twice as uncomfortable," but the feeling of more or less comfort can be experienced. If eye color is graded with a range from black to blue, we could consider this *ordinal data,* and ordinal statistics such as the median then come into play (Fig. 10-8).

The Interval Scale

The third and most commonly used level of statistical measurement is interval measurement. Actually, much ordinal data is treated as if it were

Fig. 10-7. Nominal scale

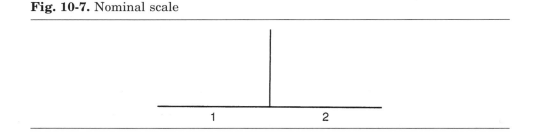

interval data. There is a great debate in statistical circles as to whether this can really be done. Interval measurements are based on absolutely equal distances between measurements, but there is no absolute zero starting point on an interval scale. Because temperatures can be measured in either Fahrenheit or Celsius and neither of these scales has an absolute zero (i.e., no temperature at all), a clinical thermometer is an interval-measuring instrument (Fig. 10-9).

The Ratio Scale

The highest level of measurement is the ratio scale (Fig. 10-10). This scale has a starting point or base of absolute zero. All subjects start at zero and travel or respond in some manner along this same scale. Length, weight, and volume are examples of ratio measurements because they start with an absolute zero (no length, no weight, or no volume). Practically speaking, nursing research is rarely of a type that deals with ratio scales.

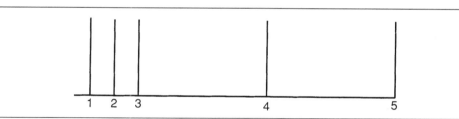

Fig. 10-8. Ordinal scale

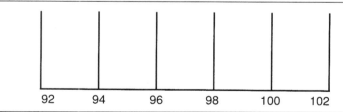

Fig. 10-9. Interval scale

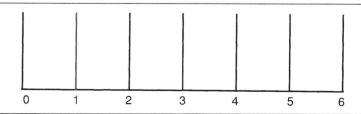

Fig. 10-10. Ratio scale

Commonly Used Statistical Tests

Regardless of the scale level used, the researcher must answer the question, "Are the differences I see caused by chance, or are other factors responsible, such as my treatment?" For example, when a researcher sees that two different groups have different means, the next task is to test the differences between the means to determine if they are significantly different statistically. Based on the level of data, the researcher selects the statistical test that is the most appropriate to determine if chance is the overriding factor. The terms *parametric statistics* and *nonparametric statistics* are associated with level of measurement of the data to be analyzed. Each of these terms refers to a different group of inferential statistical techniques. Parametric statistical techniques are intended for use with interval- and ratio-level data; nonparametric statistical techniques are intended to be used with nominal- and ordinal-level data.

Parametric Statistical Tests

The term *parametric statistics* is used to describe "a class of inferential statistics that involves (a) assumptions about the distribution of the variables, (b) the estimation of a parameter, and (c) the use of interval measures" [2]. The most frequently used parametric tests include (1) *t*-tests, (2) analysis of variance, and (3) analysis of covariance.

t-Tests

In order to determine whether the differences between the means of two different sets of scores are statistically significant, the researcher first determines whether the two samples are independent (such as in the case of an experimental and a control group) or if they are dependent (using the same group of individuals and their responses prior to and after a treatment). This must be done because there are several ways to compute the *t* statistic. If an inappropriate method is used, the researcher might obtain incorrect results in either accepting or rejecting the hypothesis.

An example of the use of the *t* statistic can be found in the study done by Warden and colleagues. This study was concerned with the effect of using mock trial procedures in developing students' ability to make clinically sound legal judgments [3]. The researchers found that students were significantly more able ($p < .05$) to make legally sound clinical judgments after being exposed to a mock trial experience. They also found that the students preferred the mock trial experience over traditional classroom presentations.

Analysis of Variance (ANOVA)

Sometimes the researcher has more than two means to test to determine if there are significant differences between them. In this instance, using the *t* statistic could be exceedingly tedious because of the number of possible permutations of the *t*-test. Also, the more individual *t*-tests conducted, the greater the possibility of what is called a *Type I error* or a *Type II error*. A Type I error means that the investigator has rejected the null hypothesis when it should be accepted. A Type II error occurs when the investigator accepts the null hypothesis when it should be rejected. Consequently, the statistical analysis of variance, or ANOVA, is often used. With this technique, it is possible to determine if there is a significant difference between several means simultaneously. The literature will report these differences as the *F*-test or the *F* ratio.

Also, when many means have been tested, the researcher will want to know exactly which means were significantly different from the other means. There are other methods, such as Sheffe's test or the Tukey HSD test, that can be applied in determining which means were significantly different from the other means.

The use of ANOVA can be found in Mercer and Ferketich's study of high- and low-risk women's perception of achieved competence in the maternal role over time [4]. They found that there was no significant difference between high-risk women and low-risk women in their perceived development of maternal competence over time (1, 4, and 8 months after birth). Thus, the researchers rejected their hypothesis that there would be a significant difference between the two groups.

Finally, researchers should be aware that ANOVA may be applied when there is more than one dependent variable to be examined. Statisticians call this *multiple analysis of variance* or MANOVA. This type of statistical analysis can become quite complex, and we urge you to have someone prepared in statistical methodology help you design such an analysis.

An example of the use of MANOVA is Foley and Stone's pilot study of stress inoculation with nursing students [5]. Students who were given training in coping with future stressors were compared with nursing students who were not given such training. The researchers identified multiple dependent variables as indicators of the extent and breadth of the impact of stress inoculation, and they found that such instruction had the potential to reduce stress and to enhance the coping skills of their subjects.

Analysis of Covariance (ANCOVA)

Frequently, because of the nature of the research setting, it is impossible for a researcher to place subjects into truly randomly assigned groups. In this case, there may be variables that confound the variable under consideration. This means that the researcher's data may or may not show significant differences unless the confounding variable or variables are accounted for.

In order to account for the confounding variable, the researcher may utilize analysis of covariance, or ANCOVA, which is also reported as an F statistic or F ratio. This procedure may be used in place of the t statistic when two groups are involved and there is no way to achieve the requirements of randomness necessary for appropriate use of the t statistic. Analysis of covariance may also be used on more than two sets of subjects or when there is more than one dependent variable.

Nonparametric Statistical Tests

The term *nonparametric statistics* is used to describe "a general class of inferential statistics that does not involve rigorous assumptions about the distribution of the critical variables; most often used when samples are small or when the data are measured on the nominal or ordinal scales" [6].

Because there are literally dozens of nonparameteric tests available, we will discuss and highlight only a few of the more commonly used statistics: (1) chi-square, (2) Mann-Whitney U, (3) Kruskal-Wallis one-way analysis of variance, and (4) Friedman two-way analysis of variance.

Chi-Square (χ^2)

Perhaps the most commonly used nonparametric statistic is the *chi-square* (χ^2) measure. This statistic can be applied to nominal or higher levels of measurement and can be used in one or more samples. Essentially, the chi-square test is used to determine if the observed frequencies of events in certain categories fall within the range of frequencies expected to fall in these categories.

For example, Byers used the chi-square statistic in her study of the relationship between infant crying and bottle feeding during aircraft descent [7]. Byers found that there was a significant difference in the amount of crying as a result of changes of air pressure in infants' ears between infants who were bottle fed during the descent and infants who were not bottle fed during the descent. Bottle-fed infants cried significantly less than their unfed counterparts.

Mann-Whitney U

A very powerful nonparametric alternative to the t-test is the *Mann-Whitney U* test. By using this statistic, a researcher can determine whether or not two groups are significantly different when the scores from two sets of data are ranked. Kalish et al. examined 320 television episodes from 28 series on prime time television from 1950 to 1980 in which nurses and nursing were portrayed [8]. Data on Nielsen ratings were used to rank the programs for level of exposure to the viewing public. A variety of statistics, including the Mann-Whitney U, were used to analyze the data. By ranking the various shows by their Neilsen ratings and applying the Mann-Whitney U, these authors concluded that technical care was the nursing action that received the highest audience exposure and that menial, non-nursing tasks had very low audience exposure.

Kruskal-Wallis One-Way Analysis of Variance

Even as parametric tests provide techniques for the analysis of variance, so do nonparametric tests. The *Kruskal-Wallis* statistic is one such test which allows for a one-way analysis of variance with ordinal data. Kalish et al. also utilized this statistic when they analyzed the world of nursing as portrayed on television [9]. The results of this study are most interesting:

> The findings showed that nurses were depicted as working in acute care settings, entering nursing for altruistic reasons, predominately acting as a resource to other health professionals, not using problem-solving and evaluation skills, deficient in administrative abilities, and remiss in providing physical comforting, engaging in expanded role activities, patient education and scholarly endeavors. Since the 1960s the trend in the quality of nurse portrayals has been downward. This has created a current crisis in communicating the world of nursing to the public via the most powerful form of mass communication, television. [10]

Friedman Two-Way Analysis of Variance by Ranks

Even as a researcher might need to use a parametric MANOVA, occasionally there is a need to use a nonparametric ANOVA. Vanbree et al. used the *Friedman two-way analysis of variance* to determine if there were significant differences in skin bruising as a result of three different subcutaneous injection techniques for administering low-dose heparin [11]. This analysis required the ranking of observations for each subject, which in this case called for ranking of sizes of bruises from the smallest to the largest. After ranking the various bruise sizes, the investigators concluded that there was no significant difference between the three subcutaneous injection techniques for administering low-dose heparin.

Correlations

Researchers are often concerned about the relationship between two variables. The relationship between two variables is measured by correlation statistics, often called measures of association. Correlation statistics range from -1.0 to $+1.0$. It is very important to note that correlations do not imply cause-and-effect relationships. Correlations that report the presence or absence of something else do not necessarily mean that one factor caused the other. For example, the correlation between houses with roofs and houses with basements probably approaches $+1.0$, but this does not mean that the presence of roofs causes basements to be present. Such a correlation would be a spurious correlation: the assumption of relationship where none really exists.

It is also important to note that a correlation of -1 is just as strong as a correlation of $+1$. The closer a correlation coefficient is to either -1 or $+1$, the stronger the relationship is between the variables being studied.

Pearson r

The commonly used parametric statistic for correlation is the Pearson product-moment correlation coefficient, otherwise known as the *Pearson r,* or more simply as r. In this test, two different sets of interval-level data are compared to determine the degree of relationship between them. Since r's range from -1 through 0 to $+1$, we can say that such sets of items are related either positively or negatively. As the correlation coefficient approaches -1 or $+1$, the items become more highly related. On the other hand, if the correlation coefficient approaches 0, we know that the items have little or no relationship.

Whether or not the degree of association is statistically significant may also be measured. That is, is the correlation coefficient a result of chance, or is the correlation really statistically significant? Jones and Thomas investigated cardiovascular changes in 148 first-time fathers while holding and interacting with their newborn infants [12]. They found that the systolic blood pressure, diastolic blood pressure, and heart rate of new fathers were significantly higher during the new fathers' verbal interaction with their newborn. The researchers also found that the diastolic blood pressure of the new fathers was positively related to the frequency of the infant crying.

Spearman Rho Correlation

As is the case in parametric statistical analysis, there is a host of nonparametric correlation techniques. One of the most common is the *Spearman rho correlation* (r_s). Researchers utilizing this statistic rank their observations of the two variables under consideration and then determine the level of relationship between them. For example, a researcher might want to test the relationship between patients' perceived level of comfort and their perception of the quality of care provided by the nursing staff in a hospital. In this instance, the patients would be given two attitude evaluation scales (one to measure each variable), and then the two scores would be ranked and a Spearman rho computed.

An example of the use of the Spearman rho can be found in the study of renal transplant patients conducted by Sutton and Murphy [13]. The researchers compared the coping scores of 40 renal transplant patients, 20 of whom had had their transplants within 23 months of measurement of their coping strategies to deal with stress and 20 other renal transplant patients who had had their transplants from 23 to 48 months before being given the same coping scale. Using the Spearman rho correlation, the investigators found that the rank orderings of coping methods according to mean degree of use were significantly correlated between the two study groups ($r_s = 0.87$). The findings of their study suggest that renal transplant patients may experience continuing stress as long as 4 years after transplant surgery.

You may also find a number of other nonparametric statistic correlation coefficients in the studies that you examine, such as Kendall's tau or Cronbach's alpha.

Partial and Multiple Correlation

Occasionally the researcher has a number of items that might be interrelated. In this instance, partial correlations can be computed. The intent of this method is to eliminate the confounding effects of one or more variables when measuring the relationships between a number of variables. This is shown as $r_{12.3}$, where variables 1 and 2 are correlated and variable 3 is eliminated mathematically.

Conversely, if you want to lump together all of the variables, this can be done by a technique called multiple correlation (symbolized by the letter *R*). O'Rourke used multiple correlation to investigate a sample of employed women's subjective appraisal of their psychological well-being (PWB), the dependent variable, and the following independent variables: (1) subjective self-reports of menstrual and nonmenstrual symptoms, (2) sociodemographic factors (age, income, ethnicity), and (3) a health factor (represented by self-reports of current health status) [14]. Results of the study indicated "a strong positive relationship between the independent variables when analyzed as a set and PWB (R = 0.86) [15]. A major finding of the study was that the presence of specific menstrual symptoms did not negatively affect PWB; rather, these women had a higher PWB than those with nonmenstrual symptoms.

In summary, we have discussed the use of descriptive and inferential statistics in data analysis and have briefly presented a few of the commonly used parametric and nonparametric statistical tests, as well as correlations.

Meta-Analysis

Meta-analysis is a quantitative data analysis strategy that examines research findings across studies: "It is the statistical analysis of a large collection of results from individual studies for the purpose of integrating the findings into a single, generalizable finding" [16]. Meta-analysis is most effective when numerous studies concerning the same variables are available, but the technique can be used when only a few studies have been done.

For example, Perez-Escamilla and colleagues explored the relationship between breast-feeding policies in maternity wards and breast-feeding success by using meta-analytical techniques [17]. The authors reviewed 65 studies, in English or Spanish, published between 1951 and 1991 concerning the relationship between maternity ward practices and lactation success that would fit a rigorous, predefined set of criteria for inclusion in the study. The researchers identified 18 studies in this body of literature that met the inclusion criteria. Using meta-analytical techniques, the researchers found that hospital based breast-feeding interventions and the elimination of commercial discharge packs can have a beneficial impact on lactation success, especially in primiparas.

The Use of Computers and Calculators in Quantitative Data Analysis

With the advent of computers and hand-held calculators, statistical analysis of quantitative data has become increasingly sophisticated. This is because many calculations that required hours or days of work when figured by hand or on mechanical calculators can now be done in seconds or minutes by the computer or hand calculator, with far greater accuracy and fewer mistakes.

Anyone who is serious about research and statistics should acquire a hand calculator. These range from simple, inexpensive devices to fairly expensive, programmable machines. For ease of computation, there are a number of calculators designed to compute the mean, standard deviation, and variance. We strongly urge that any hand calculator you purchase have these features.

Most researchers also have access to one or more computers. These technologically complex machines may be intimidating to a beginning researcher. Remember, the computer is simply a tool that one uses for data analysis.

Computers use a number of "languages." FORTRAN, BASIC, APL, COBOL, C, and Pascal are a few of the commonly used languages. Each of these languages enhances human-machine interaction and aids in data analysis. It is not necessary, however, for a researcher to know a specific computer language to use the machine. Usually, there are teams of consultants who are willing to help the researcher and many prewritten statistical packages are widely available. One of the easiest and most powerful set of programs to use is Minitab. Another common statistical package is the Statistical Package for the Social Sciences (SPSS). Yet another very useful set of programs is the Biomedical Data Package (BMDP). Finally, the data analysis package Statistical Analysis System (SAS) is also available. Although these statistical packages were written for mainframe or large computers, some have been modified for use on smaller personal computers. It is important to note that there are an increasing number of sophisticated statistical packages designed to operate on a personal computer.

All researchers would do well to remember the saying "garbage in, garbage out." The computer can only act on the data given it. If research is poorly designed or organized, the finest computer in the world will not provide a valid statistical analysis.

There is a great temptation to subject all data to computer analysis just because of the availability of the machine. Frequently, when the number of subjects is small and the statistical computation is fairly simple, it is faster and cheaper to do one's calculations with a hand calculator.

Qualitative Data Analysis

Data for qualitative studies "are usually in the form of narrative text derived from transcribed interviews, written descriptions of observations in field notes and reflections on the dynamics of the setting in the researcher's diary" [18]. As a result, qualitative studies have voluminous amounts of data that often makes data analysis more difficult and time-consuming than in quantitative studies. In qualitative research, data collection and analysis occur simultaneously, as the researcher continually interprets data from the outset of the study. Data are coded to facilitate the identification and analysis of meaningful categories inherent in the data. The analysis of qualitative data requires a great deal of mulling over of the data before the researcher can draw conclusions and communicate the findings. The following discussion of published studies that exemplify the major qualitative approaches is intended to give you an idea of how data are collected, analyzed, and interpreted in qualitative studies.

Phenomenology

Phenomenology was previously defined as the study of human experience. A data analysis technique used in phenomenologic studies involves data from interviews with study subjects to discover themes or categories of experiences as viewed from the subjects' perspective. For example, McLain used a phenomenologic approach to determine nurse–physician interactions between nine family nurse practitioners and their physician partners [19]. Participants were interviewed both separately and together about their practice relationships. An analysis of emergent themes in the data revealed the existence of distorted communication and nonmeaningful interaction. Elements that could contribute to a successful collaborative practice included "a willingness to move beyond basic information exchange in nurse/physician interactions, the willingness and ability to challenge distortions and assumptions in the relationship, and a belief system based on critical self-reflection" [20]. Additionally, Baumann used the phenomenologic approach to determine the meaning of being homeless as described by 15 homeless women with dependent children [21]. Participants were interviewed and a three-level phenomenologic method was utilized to interpret the meaning of being homeless. Baumann found that the meaning of being homeless used the metaphor of an individual being caught in a whirlpool that only spirals downward and over which the individual has no control.

Grounded Theory

Grounded theory uses the steps of the research process simultaneously. The researcher observes, collects data, organizes the data, and develops theory all at the same time. The grounded theory researcher uses the constant comparative method of data analysis in which every piece of data is compared to every other datum (an individual data item). In her study of caregiving of relatives with Alzheimer's dementia, Wilson used the constant comparative method to explore the dilemmas faced by family members trying to cope with a relative with Alzheimer's dementia [22]. She used the computer program *Ethnograph* to analyze the verbal data collected from 20 in-depth face-to-face interviews with family caregivers. Findings indicated that caregivers had only negative choices in caring for their afflicted relative at home; that is, no matter which choice was made, there were undesirable consequences for the caregiver.

In another study of homeless women, Montgomery used grounded theory methodology to examine how these women overcame the problems of being homeless [23]. She interviewed seven women and found that homelessness, for these women, was a temporary condition, which resulted from an attempt to break away from an abusive or oppressive situation and to move toward a better life.

Ethnography

Ethnographic research has its roots in the discipline of anthropology. The ethnographer's purpose is to study cultures by using systematic observation. This type of study allows the researcher to gain knowledge and insights concerning the lifeways or patterns of particular cultures. Ethnographic research can prove to be extremely valuable in gaining knowledge of folk medicine practiced by a cultural group in order to understand how to improve health care practices by members of the group. Such a study was done by Cheon-Klessig et al. when they studied the folk medical practices of Hmong refugees residing in the United States [24]. The researchers used a variety of data-gathering techniques including "unstructured interviews, informal conversations, written documents, and participation in events . . ." to gather "data that were used to identify the general health care patterns and folk medicine usage in this group of Hmong refugees. . . ." [25].

The researchers found that the Hmong used a variety of herbal medicines and that householders often grew some of the plants used. The researchers also found that herbalists were called on to treat ill individuals and that the Hmong called in shamans to diagnose and treat diseases. Further, they found that many Hmong were reluctant to use U.S. health care practices because they felt that surgery and blood tests had the potential for great harm both in the present and in the afterlife. In this instance, there is a great conflict between the beliefs of the Hmong and the U.S. medical system. As a result, many Hmong either do not use the U.S. health care system or may not comply with treatments if the treatments are in conflict with their traditional medical beliefs.

In another study that identified themes in managing culturally defined illness in Cambodian refugee families, Frye and D'Avanzo investigated family managed stress-related symptoms resulting from traumatic experiences which took place during the Khmer Rouge regime in Cambodia [26]. The researchers interviewed 120 Cambodian refugee women and found that many individuals in the Cambodian refugee community suffered from depression, which was called *koucharang* or "thinking too much." The researchers identified two cultural themes: withdrawal by the affected individual and the sheltering (speaking softly and positively) of the affected individual by the family.

The Use of Computers in Qualitative Data Analysis

Qualitative data may also be analyzed using computers. There are a number of programs mentioned in the qualitative data analysis literature and programs such as *Ethnograph, Nud*ist, Martin,* or *Gator.* These programs can analyze verbal data to find themes or problem areas that are shared by subjects. Occasionally, the use of a word-processing program that displays word counts aids the qualitative researcher in finding common themes or ideas.

This chapter presented a few basic ideas about data analysis. Any researcher who wishes to deal in greater depth in either quantitative or qualitative strategies is strongly urged to take one or more courses that feature the appropriate data-gathering and analysis techniques.

The Workbook Activities for this chapter will help to evaluate your understanding of the material related to data analysis.

References

1. Cohen, B. 1984. "Florence Nightingale." *Scientific American,* 250 (March): 128–137.

2. Polit, D. F., and B. P. Hungler. *Nursing Research: Principles and Methods,* 5th ed. Philadelphia: J. B. Lippincott, 1995, pp. 648–649.

3. Warden, S., et al. 1994. "The Effect of a Mock Trial on Nursing Students' Ability to Make Clinically Sound Legal Judgements." *Nurse Educator,* 19 (May–June): 18–22.

4. Mercer, R., and S. L. Ferketich. 1994. "Predictors of Maternal Role Competence by Risk Status." *Nursing Research,* 43 (January–February): 38–43.

5. Foley, J., and G. L. Stone. 1988. "Stress Inoculation with Nursing Students." *Western Journal of Nursing Research,* 10 (August): 435–448.

6. Polit and Hungler, *Nursing Research,* p. 647.

7. Byers, P. H. 1986. "Infant Crying During Aircraft Descent." *Nursing Research,* 35 (September–October): 260–262.

8. Kalish, P. A., B. J. Kalish, and J. Clinton. 1982. "The World of Nursing on Prime Time Television, 1950 to 1980." *Nursing Research,* 31 (November–December): 358–363.

9. Ibid.

10. Ibid., p. 358.

11. Vanbree, N., A. D. Hollerbach, and G. P. Brooks. 1984. "Clinical Evaluation of Three Techniques for Administering Low-Dose Heparin." *Nursing Research,* 33 (January–February): 15–19.

12. Jones, L. C., and S. A. Thomas. 1989. "New Fathers' Blood Pressure and Heart Rate: Relationships to Interaction with Their Newborn Infants." *Nursing Research,* 38 (July–August): 237–241.

13. Sutton, T. D., and S. P. Murphy. 1989. "Stressors and Patterns of Coping in Renal Transplant Patients." *Nursing Research,* 38 (January–February): 46–49.

14. O'Rourke, M. W. 1983. "Subjective Appraisal of Psychological Well Being and Self-Reports of Menstrual and Non-Menstrual Symptomatology in Employed Women." *Nursing Research,* 32 (September–October): 288–292.

15. Ibid., p. 288.

16. Lynn, M. R. 1989. "Meta-Analysis: Appropriate Tool for the Integration of Nursing Research?" *Nursing Research,* 38 (5): 302.

17. Perez-Escamilla, R., et al. 1994. "Infant Feeding Policies in Maternity Wards and Their Effect on Breast-Feeding Success: An Overview." *American Journal of Public Health,* 84 (January): 89–97.

18. Field, P. A., and J. M. Morse. 1985. *Nursing Research: The Application of Qualitative Approaches.* Rockville, MD: Aspen, p. 96.

19. McLain, B. R. 1988. "Collaborative Practice: A Critical Theory Perspective." *Research in Nursing and Health,* 11 (December): 391–398.

20. Ibid., p. 391.

21. Baumann, S. L. 1993. "The Meaning of Being Homeless." *Scholarly Inquiry for Nursing Practice,* 7: 59–69.

22. Wilson, H. S. 1989. "Family Caregiving for a Relative with Alzheimer's Dementia: Coping with Negative Choices." *Nursing Research,* 38 (March–April): 94–98.
23. Montgomery, C. 1994. "Swimming Upstream: The Strengths of Women Who Survive Homelessness." *Advances in Nursing Science,* 16: 34–45.
24. Cheon-Klessig, Y., D. Camilleri, B. J. McElmurry, and V. M. Ohlson. 1988. "Folk Medicine in the Health Practice of Hmong Refugees." *Western Journal of Nursing Research,* 10: 647–660.
25. Ibid., p. 650.
26. Frye, B., and C. D'Avanzo. 1994. "Themes in Managing Culturally Defined Illness in the Cambodian Refugee Family." *Journal of Community Health Nursing,* 11: 89–98.

Bibliography and Suggested Readings

Baumann, S. L. 1993. "The Meaning of Being Homeless." *Scholarly Inquiry for Nursing Practice,* 7: 59–69.

Brent, E. 1984. "Qualitative Computing: Approaches and Issues." *Qualitative Sociology,* 7 (Spring–Summer): 360–365.

Byers, P. H. 1986. "Infant Crying During Aircraft Descent." *Nursing Research,* 35 (September–October): 260–262.

Cheon-Klessig, Y., D. Camilleri, B. J. McElmurry, and V. M. Ohlson. 1988. "Folk Medicine in the Health Practice of Hmong Refugees." *Western Journal of Nursing Research,* 10: 647–660.

Cochran, S., and J. Holliman. 1974. *Cheat Sheet for Stat.* Commerce: TX: Authors.

Cohen, Bernard. 1984. "Florence Nightingale." *Scientific American,* 250 (March): 128–137.

Field, P. A., and J. M. Morse. 1985. *Nursing Research: The Application of Qualitative Approaches.* Rockville, MD: Aspen.

Foley, J., and G. L. Stone. 1988. "Stress Inoculation with Nursing Students." *Western Journal of Nursing Research,* 10 (August): 435–448.

Frye, B., and C. D'Avanzo. 1994. "Themes in Managing Culturally Defined Illness in the Cambodian Refugee Family." *Journal of Community Health Nursing,* 11: 89–98.

Jones, C., and S. A. Thomas. 1989. "New Fathers' Blood Pressure and Heart Rate: Relationships to Interaction with Their Newborn Infants." *Nursing Research,* 38 (July–August): 237–241.

Kalish, P. A., B. J. Kalish, and J. Clinton. 1982. "The World of Nursing on Prime Time Television, 1950 to 1980." *Nursing Research,* 31 (November–December): 358–363.

Lynn, M. R. 1989. "Meta-Analysis: Appropriate Tool for the Integration of Nursing Research?" *Nursing Research,* 38 (September–October): 302–305.

McLain, B. R. 1988. "Collaborative Practice: A Critical Theory Perspective." *Research in Nursing and Health,* 11 (December): 391–398.

Mercer, R., and S. L. Ferketich. 1994. "Predictors of Maternal Role Competence by Risk Status." *Nursing Research,* 43 (January–February): 38–43.

Montgomery, C. 1994. "Swimming Upstream: The Strengths of Women Who Survive Homelessness." *Advances in Nursing Science,* 16: 34–45.

Mullen, B., and R. Rosenthal. 1985. *Basic Meta-Analysis Procedures and Programs.* Hillsdale, NJ: Lawrence Erlbaum Associates.

Munhall, P., and C. O. Boyd. 1993. *Nursing Research: A Qualitative Perspective,* 2nd ed. New York: National League for Nursing Press.

Munro, B. H., M. A. Visintainer, and E. B. Page. 1986. *Statistical Methods for Health Care Research.* Philadelphia: J. B. Lippincott.

O'Rourke, M. W. 1983. "Subjective Appraisal of Psychological Well Being and Self-Reports of Menstrual and Non-Menstrual Symptomatology in Employed Women." *Nursing Research,* 32 (September–October): 288–292.

Perez-Escamilla, R., E. Pollitt, B. Lönnerdahl, and K. G. Dewey. 1994. "Infant Feeding Policies in Maternity Wards and Their Effect on Breast-Feeding Success: An Overview." *American Journal of Public Health,* 84 (January): 89–97.

Polit, D. F., and B. P. Hungler. 1995. *Nursing Research: Principles and Methods.* 5th ed. Philadelphia: J. B. Lippincott, pp. 648–649.

Polkington, D. 1983. *Methodology for Human Sciences.* Albany, NY: State University of New York Press.

Seidel, J. V., and J. A. Clark. 1984. "The Ethnograph: A Computer Program for the Analysis of Qualitative Data." *Qualitative Sociology,* 7 (Spring–Summer): 110–125.

Siegal, S. 1956. *Nonparametric Statistics for the Behavioral Sciences.* New York: McGraw-Hill.

Spradley, J. P. 1979. *The Ethnographic Interview.* New York: Holt, Rinehart and Winston.

Starter, B., Ed. 1988. *Paths to Knowledge: Innovative Research Methods for Nursing.* New York: National League for Nursing.

Stone, P. J., et al. 1966. *The General Inquirer: A Computer Approach to Content Analysis.* Cambridge, MA: MIT Press.

Sutton, T. D., and P. S. Murphy. 1989. "Stressors and Patterns of Coping in Renal Transplant Patients." *Nursing Research,* 38 (September–October): 46–49.

Vanbree, N., A. D. Hollerbach, and G. P. Brooks. 1984. "Clinical Evaluation of Three Techniques of Administering Heparin." *Nursing Research,* 33 (January–February): 15–19.

Warden, S., et al. 1994. "The Effect of a Mock Trial on Nursing Students'

Ability to Make Clinically Sound Legal Judgements." *Nurse Educator,* 19 (May–June): 18–22.

Wilson, H. S. 1989. "Family Caregiving for a Relative with Alzheimer's Dementia: Coping with Negative Choices." *Nursing Research,* 38 (March–April): 94–98.

11 Communicating the Research Results

Objectives

When you have finished reading this chapter you should be able to:

1. Discuss the importance of careful interpretation of research findings
2. Describe three ways of communicating research results
3. Identify the components of a written research report
4. Discuss the purposes for preparing an abstract of a research study

---

Interpreting the Findings
Writing the Research Report
   Purposes and Characteristics
   Format
   Guidelines for Writing a Research Report
Preparing an Abstract of the Study
A Note on Publication
A Note on Presentations

In the previous chapters we presented material related to Stage I of a research study, the *planning stage*. The first six steps of the research process were discussed:

1. Statement of the problem
2. Review of related literature
3. Statement of the purpose of the study
4. Definition of the terms
5. Plan for data collection
6. Plan for data analysis

During the planning stage, the investigator develops a research proposal and provides specific information on the first six steps in the research process.

In Stage II of the research study, the *implementation stage,* the investigator puts the research plan into action by collecting the data and analyzing it in order to determine the study's results.

In Stage III of the research study, the *communication stage,* the investigator interprets the findings, formulates conclusions for the study, and communicates these in the written report of the completed study so that others may share the knowledge. This is the task we will discuss in this chapter.

Interpreting the Findings

The data collected in carrying out the study now need to be given meaning by the investigator, who interprets them in terms of the study's purpose. If the purpose of the study was to describe certain variables, then meaningful descriptions are indicated. If the study asked a question, the findings should be interpreted to answer this question. If a hypothesis was tested, the study findings should be interpreted as support or rejection of the hypothesis.

Data interpretation is a subjective process; the investigator must be extremely careful not to interpret beyond what the data indicate and must relate conclusions to the study purpose.

Researchers are often hesitant to report negative results of their studies. These are results that contradict the theoretical or conceptual framework or fail to support the study's hypothesis. In a well-designed research study, however, such scientifically derived results can add as much to the existing body of scientific knowledge as the results of studies where the results expected by the investigator are produced.

Sometimes a study has important and unexpected findings not related to the original purpose of the study. These are called *serendipitous findings.* The investigator needs to be aware of the possible existence of such findings and the importance of interpreting and reporting them. In order to add to existing knowledge, the investigator should also be prepared to relate the study findings to other studies in the same area. All studies have their own limitations over which the investigator has no control. These limitations and their effect on the interpretation of the data should be discussed.

Finally, because the investigator is the expert on this study, interpretation of the data should result in a discussion of implications for the practice or profession of nursing, and recommendations for further research.

Writing the Research Report

As a final step in the research process, the investigator writes a research report to make the results available and known to others.

Purposes and Characteristics

A research report has several purposes. It may communicate the research results to other investigators, in which case the report should communicate the purpose, procedures, and findings in sufficient detail so that another investigator could replicate the study. In addition, consumers of nursing research need to become aware of reported research so that they may critically analyze the findings and use them in practice.

Format

A research report should be objective, concise, and scholarly in spelling, grammar, and punctuation. A dictionary and a style manual should be used when writing the report. Individual authors such as Campbell and Turabian and associations such as the American Psychological Association and the Modern Language Association have developed style manuals. Some journals have developed their own style sheets, available upon request; or the required format may be found on the journal's front or back cover.

Research reports vary from detailed reports to abridged versions for publication. The following format is suggested for preparing a detailed report.

Guidelines for Writing a Research Report

The report is divided into three major parts: (1) preliminary materials, (2) main body (text) of the report, and (3) reference materials. Each major part consists of several sections, represented in the following outline:

I. Preliminary materials
   A. Title page
   B. Table of contents
   C. List of illustrations (figures)
   D. List of tables
   E. Preface or acknowledgment (if any)
II. Main body (text) of the report
   A. Introduction
      1. Statement of the problem
      2. Review of related literature, including conceptual or theoretical framework if appropriate
      3. Purpose of the study
      4. Definition of terms
      5. Assumptions of the study
   B. Methodology
      1. Research approach
      2. Study subjects

      3. Techniques for data collection
      4. Procedures
      5. Limitations of the study
    C. Findings
      1. Data are reported and their meaning discussed.
      2. Tables, graphs, figures are included and discussed in the text.
    D. Discussion
      1. Interpretation of findings and conclusions
      2. Comparison of findings with those of other investigations
      3. Implications for nursing
      4. Recommendations for further study
    E. Summary
      1. Brief restatement of problem
      2. Brief review of procedures, major conclusions, and recommendations
III. Reference materials
    A. Bibliography
    B. Appendix(es) (if any)
    C. Glossary (if any)

The title of the report should reflect the relationship between the study variables and the study population.

In the findings section of the report, the investigator reports and analyzes the data objectively. Appropriate statistical information is presented and discussed. Each table, graph, or figure used to summarize the data is discussed in the text and should be placed as close as possible to the first text reference to it.

In the discussion section of the report, data are interpreted according to the study's purpose and the study results are compared with results obtained in other studies. The investigator then formulates implications for nursing and recommendations for further research.

In the summary section, the study's most important aspects are presented in a brief restatement of the problem and the purpose of the study. A brief review of the data collection procedures and a brief summary of the major conclusions and recommendations are also included.

The bibliography section should list all the sources used to write the report. The appendix section includes materials especially designed for the study, such as cover letters or questionnaires. The raw data from the study may be included in this section.

Preparing an Abstract of the Study

An abstract is a concise summary of the study. Although abstracts vary in length, depending on the purpose of the study, they are usually limited to 150 to 200 words.

Researchers write abstracts for several purposes. When placed at the beginning of a research report published as a journal article, an abstract presents an overview of the research problem and the methodology used, and an interpretation of the results of the study. This brief overview permits the reader to decide whether or not to read the complete article. Abstracts are also written in response to a call for papers for professional meetings, primarily to determine if the study topic is relevant to the sessions being planned for the meeting [1].

A Note on Publication

If you decide to write an article for a professional journal based on your research, it is advisable to look over current publications in the area of your study to see where it will have the best chances of being accepted, then write a query letter to the editor of the publication to which you would like to submit your article. This letter should include a brief statement of your own background relevant to your article, a brief description of the article you plan to write, and an outline of the article if possible. You should also request publication guidelines in your letter.

Although it is permissible to submit query letters to several publication editors at the same time, journal stipulations and professional ethics dictate that the manuscript for the final article be submitted to only one publication at a time [2]. The term *refereed* is used in connection with submitting manuscripts for publication. The referee system is a process of having three or more experts independently review and judge the merits of the manuscript before making a decision about publication:

> The implication is that refereed nursing journals are the source and repository of reliable, valid clinical papers through which the refinement of professional practice occurs—and hence, bring higher prestige to authors appearing in them than nonrefereed journals do. [3]

A final word: Do not become discouraged if your first query letter fails to elicit a positive response. Keep on trying with other journals.

A Note on Presentations

Meetings of professional organizations give researchers an opportunity to present their findings before an audience of their peers. These presentations may range from formal to informal sessions. In any case, certain basic guidelines should be followed.

Your paper should be prepared well in advance of the presentation. Although organizations usually request an abstract before accepting a paper, the preparation of an abstract may not mean that the entire paper is ready.

It is embarrassing for both audience and presenter when it is obvious that the presenter has not mastered the information to be presented.

Be sure that any audiovisual materials that you plan to use are appropriate and that the devices needed to present them are available. If the organization does not indicate whether the necessary equipment is available, you should contact the organizers or bring your own.

Be sure that your audiovisual materials are properly arranged and organized. Slides that must be viewed upside-down or backward, or overhead projection materials that are too small to read from the back of the room, lead audiences to boredom and presenters to frustration.

Many organizations now provide opportunities for researchers to present at poster sessions. These presentations are more informal than the presentation of a paper, but posters should be well organized and interestingly presented. Remember, the information that you have to give is important, and the amount of time and effort spent in research can be negated or trivialized if the materials are poorly organized.

The Workbook Activities are designed to help you evaluate your understanding of principles and procedures related to the material in this chapter.

References

1. Fuller, E. 1983. "Preparing an Abstract of a Nursing Study." *Nursing Research,* 32 (September–October): 316–317.
2. Brosnan, J., and A. Kovalsky. 1980. "Perishing while Publishing." *Nursing Outlook,* 28 (November): 688.
3. Clayton, B. C., and K. Boyle. 1981. "The Refereed Journal: Prestige in Professional Publication." *Nursing Outlook,* 29 (September): 531.

Bibliography and Suggested Readings

Benjaminson, P. 1992. *Publish Without Perishing: A Practical Handbook for Academic Authors.* Washington, D.C.: NEA Professional Library.

Brosnan, J., and A. Kovalsky. 1980. "Perishing while Publishing." *Nursing Outlook,* 28 (November): 688.

Clayton, B. C., and K. Boyle. 1981. "The Refereed Journal: Prestige in Professional Publication." *Nursing Outlook,* 29 (September): 531–534.

Field, P. A., and J. M. Morse. 1985. *Nursing Research: The Application of Qualitative Approaches.* Rockville, MD: Aspen.

Fuller, E. 1983. "Preparing an Abstract of a Nursing Study." *Nursing Research,* 32 (September–October): 316–317.

Gay, L. R. 1992. *Educational Research: Competencies for Analysis and Application,* 4th ed. Columbus, OH: Charles E. Merrill.

Hagemaster, J. N., and K. M. Kerrins. 1984. "Six Easy Steps to Publishing." *Nursing Educator,* 9: 32–34.

Luey, B. 1990. *Handbook for Academic Authors.* rev. ed. Cambridge, NY: Cambridge University Press.

Moxley, J. M. 1992. *Publish Don't Perish: A Scholar's Guide to Academic Writing and Publishing.* Westport, CT: Greenwood Press.

Moxley, J. M., Ed. 1992. *Writing and Publishing for Academic Authors.* Lanham, MD: University Press of America.

Part III

Applying the Results of Scientific Inquiry to Nursing Practice

The material in Part III is designed to acquaint you with principles and techniques for utilizing the results of scientific inquiry to improve nursing practice. Chapter 12 discusses current issues regarding the utilization of research knowledge and provides techniques for participating in the process of using valid research findings to improve patient care.

12 Utilizing the Results of Research

Objectives

When you have finished reading this chapter you should be able to:

1. Define research utilization
2. Explain the relationship between the conduct of research and the utilization of research
3. Discuss at least three issues related to utilizing research findings in clinical practice
4. Identify three major federally funded utilization projects
5. Describe the research utilization process
6. Identify the role of the baccalaureate prepared nurse in the research utilization process

---

Relationship of Research Conduct and Research Utilization
Issues in Research Utilization
Major Utilization Projects
    Regional Program for Nursing Research and Development (WICHE) Project
    Nursing Child Assessment Satellite Training (NCAST) Projects
    Conduct and Utilization of Research in Nursing (CURN) Project
Research Utilization in the 1990s
The Research Utilization Process

In previous chapters we have presented material related to the steps involved in the first three stages of the research process. In Stage I, the planning stage, a research proposal developed by the investigator addresses the first five steps of the research process. In Stage II, the implementation stage, the researcher activates the research plan by collecting data and analyzing them in order to determine the study's results. In Stage III, the communication stage, the investigator interprets and communicates the findings, either in a written or verbal report or in publications. Finally, efforts are directed toward utilizing the results of research to improve nursing practice. The material in this chapter is designed to acquaint you with current issues regarding the utilization of research knowledge, and the processes involved in translating valid research-based findings into the delivery of improved patient care.

Relationship of Research Conduct and Research Utilization

Research conduct and research utilization are interdependent processes, both help to further the development of a scientific basis of practice for nursing: "The purpose of research is to identify and refine solutions to problems through the generation of new knowledge, while the purpose of research utilization is to get the new solutions used for the good of society. Neither process taken alone is sufficient to meet the needs of society" [1].

Research conduct is directed toward producing knowledge that is generalizable beyond the study population, whereas research utilization is directed at transferring this specific research-based knowledge into actual practice. The term *research utilization* has a simple, straightforward meaning: to use the methods and products of research. "In the most general sense, research methods and products are used to expand knowledge and to verify or change practice" [2]. Research utilization may mean changing a current practice by developing or updating already existing protocols for nursing care so they are based on available scientific research. It may also mean evaluating a research-based protocol already in use to see if it is being successfully implemented in the clinical setting [3].

The potential gap between the scientific identification of solutions to problems through research conduct and the utilization of these solutions is exemplified in the following:

> Merely imparting or transmitting the results of research is usually insufficient. For example, as a guide for future planning, one mental hospital undertook to study the effect of the furnishings in dayrooms on patients' socialization patterns. One dayroom was furnished with Swedish Modern furniture and the other with Early American. Observations over a considerable period of time showed that the patients constantly favored the room with Swedish Modern furniture; they found it more congenial and comfortable. However, when the hospital needed

new furniture, the staff responsible for requisitioning new supplies paid
no attention to the results of this study. They ordered what they had
always ordered, Early American furniture. . . . Here was research that
was not utilized. Unfortunately, this is not an uncommon kind of occurrence. [4]

As the nursing profession has come to value nursing research, the research base for nursing practice has increased over the past few years.
However, there has been a major time lag between the knowledge generated by research and its utilization for improving nursing practice. In a
national survey reported by Lindeman in 1975, 15 priorities were established that were considered to have the most significant potential for impact on patients' welfare. "In the decade since those priorities were published, research has made strides in most of these areas. The priority item,
'Determine means for greater utilization of research in practice,' however,
has not enjoyed as much success as the other priorities" [5]. In the 20 years
since Lindeman's survey, the literature has consistently reflected widespread agreement among nursing professionals that nursing must establish itself as a research-based profession with a strong scientific basis for
practice.

Nursing is not alone in its concern with translating research findings
into practice:

> Knowledge is expanding rapidly in many disciplines, but its use does
> not seem to be keeping pace . . . Why some findings require much longer
> to implement than others is not clearly understood. Historical events,
> attitudes toward the researcher and research in general, and the neces-
> sity with some innovations to change attitudes and values before the
> findings can be accepted and utilized seem to influence the time re-
> quired. [6]

Issues in Research Utilization

Issues related to the generation of nursing research for utilization in practice fall into several categories: those associated with the dissemination
of valid findings to receptive users; those related to the varied contexts in
which nurse scientists and nurse clinicians work; and those related to the
actual utilization of the findings in practice, specifically to determining
who is expected to assume responsibility for carrying out the activities
necessary to transfer research-based knowledge into research-based practice.

In 1972 Diers identified three barriers related to the dissemination and
utilization of the findings of nursing research: (1) finding the findings;
(2) finding the good findings—that is, those findings that meet the criteria
for quality research and significance to nursing practice; and (3) imple-

menting the good findings [7]. In 1978, Krueger and colleagues described the need for a systematic analysis of research studies: "Nursing research must be made accessible by systematic identification, evaluation, and collation of generalizations" [8]. These authors asserted that this is primarily the responsibility of experts in nursing practice and research—not the individual nurse—and that the results should be made available through published indexes and nursing journals.

With the relatively recent advent of computer access to data bases, the issue of locating research findings is no longer as significant an issue as it was even a decade ago.

A related research dissemination issue concerns the process of disseminating research to nurses practicing in clinical areas. Should these nurses be expected to read original research reports rather than reviews of research, which summarize research findings? Do such summaries of original research discourage the professional responsibility that each nurse should have to read original research, or do the summaries actually promote an understanding of research and facilitate transfer of research-based results? Should it be the responsibility of the original investigator to write research reports in two formats—one for the scientific community and one for the much larger group of nurses who lack the academic preparation to read and understand original research reports? [9]. Although current opinion regarding the answers to these questions varies within nursing's scientific community, all agree that research findings must be disseminated to clinicians in such a way that the current gap between the generation of research findings and their use in practice can be narrowed.

A second issue in the clinical utilization of scientific nursing knowledge is related to the varied contexts in which nurse clinicians and nurse scientists work and their different goals. Nurse clinicians provide individualized patient and family care, which focuses on individual differences. Nurse scientists attempt to minimize the impact of individual differences in order to generalize results to larger groups to produce a science of nursing [10].

A third issue in research utilization is related to the actual utilization of the findings in practice: Who is expected to assume responsibility for carrying out the activities necessary to transfer research-based knowledge into research-based nursing practice? Specifically, should individual practicing staff nurses be expected to make usable changes in their practice on the basis of knowledge gained through research, or is this an organizational responsibility?

Throughout the past 20 years, several surveys have shown that staff nurses were relatively unaware of research findings and that the use of research in their practice has been limited. Ketefian's 1975 investigation of the impact of nursing research on nursing practice was designed to determine the extent to which a series of research findings on the mode of temperature determination were being used by nursing practitioners. Her conclusions demonstrated the major gap between knowledge and practice: "A clear picture emerged: The practitioner either was totally unaware of the research literature relative to her practice, or, if she was aware of it, was unable to relate to it or utilize it" [11].

Kirchhoff's 1982 report of a national survey of critical care nurses' coronary precautions revealed that the awareness of published studies had not significantly changed practice [12].

In a 1994 study, 212 medical-surgical nurses employed in 6 hospitals were asked to self-report their use of the methods and products of research and to identify their attitudes toward the use of research-based knowledge in clinical practice. Respondents rated research-based practice change as the most difficult, indicating their perception of the difficulty involved in changing practice based on research findings. Although they "delegate the translation of research findings into usable formats to educators and researchers," most subjects reported they were interested in learning how to develop research-based patient protocols [13].

Although the individual practicing nurse is expected to use valid research findings to provide scientifically based patient care, it may not be feasible to expect that each practicing nurse will be able to identify, translate, and use relevant research findings in practice [14].

The majority of practicing nurses have been prepared at the associate degree or diploma level. It is at the baccalaureate level, however, that nurses are exposed to formal nursing research content designed to prepare them to evaluate research studies critically, which is the initial step in the utilization process. Baccalaureate research courses may not be designed to teach the research utilization process. Additionally, there are many baccalaureate-prepared nurses who graduated before the relatively recent introduction of research into nursing curriculums.

It is obvious that the individual practicing nurse is expected to use valid research findings to provide scientifically sound patient care. However, it may not be feasible to expect that each practicing nurse will be able to identify, translate, and use relevant research findings in practice:

> The setting for nursing practice plays a large role in whether or not research is perceived as important to practice. For staff members to value research, the importance of research in improving the quality of nursing care would have to be reinforced by administration; members of the staff would need to have time off to attend nursing conferences, and a small library with current journals would be made available for perusal in spare moments. When few resources are available and when nurses have no voice in policy for the delivery of care, creativity and testing of ideas are rarely visible. There is no incentive for "bucking the system"; and certainly there are few rewards. [15]

At this stage in the progress of utilization of research-based knowledge in practice settings, it would seem that appropriate and effective utilization can be best accomplished through a collaborative process involving the efforts of clinicians, administrators, researchers, and educators.

Clinicians often begin the process by identifying problem areas, and they are the ultimate users of research-based knowledge. Administrators must facilitate various types of research activities in a number of ways, ranging from providing open encouragement of staff interest, to securing the necessary support and resources.

Researchers should include implications for nursing practice in their reports, and make concrete and practical suggestions for formatting their findings for use in the clinical setting. Educators should assist nurses through the systematic review of research, both to help extract research-based knowledge that has validity and relevance for practice and to translate the criteria for evaluating research findings into terms that clinicians can use [16].

A 1990 literature review identified techniques to facilitate nursing research utilization. The review reinforced the collaborative nature of research utilization activities: "the review support[ed] the need for the concerted efforts of the entire profession to implement research findings into practice" [17].

Major Utilization Projects

Beginning in the 1970s, three large-scale utilization projects received grant support from the Division of Nursing at the federal level: (1) the Regional Program for Nursing Research and Development Project carried out by staff members of the Western Interstate Commission for Higher Education (WICHE); (2) the Nursing Child Assessment Satellite Training Projects (NCAST); and (3) the Conduct and Utilization of Research in Nursing (CURN) Project conducted under the auspices of the Michigan Nurses' Association. All of these projects were designed to bridge the gap between the conduct of research and its utilization in clinical practice.

Regional Program for Nursing Research and Development (WICHE) Project

With the goal of increasing the quantity, quality, and use of nursing research in the western United States, WICHE, headquartered in Boulder, Colorado, was funded in 1971 by the Division of Nursing. The primary thrust of the program was "to support collaborative research endeavors among nurses from different settings and by both prepared and potential nurse researchers." An additional grant, funded in 1974, enabled the project staff to begin "the first large-scale structured approach to using valid clinical nursing research findings in the patient care setting" [18].

Three types of research groups for nurses were developed during the project: nontargeted groups, targeted groups, and utilization groups. Each group represented a different approach to nursing research.

> The goal of non-targeted research was the generation of research hypotheses from care settings by nurses caring for patients. In contrast to the single investigator–single institution approach that characterized nursing research in the 1960s, the non-targeted, regional approach brings groups of nurses with different skills and backgrounds together. . . . The long-term goal of targeted research is to develop valid and reliable instruments, composed of indicators known to be related to change in health status or level for the purpose of assessing quality of nursing care. [19]

The goal of the utilization groups was to help nurses to "locate, evaluate, choose and make plans for using research findings to change the care they provide to patients" [20]. Nurses from the western region met in a series of workshops to develop plans for basing changes in nursing care in their own settings on research findings. Dracup and Breu's article "Using Nursing Research Findings to Meet the Needs of Grieving Spouses" (1978) is a report of their experiences with a utilization project in a coronary care setting developed at one of the regional workshops. In 1978, Krueger and colleagues provided the following recommendation regarding this large-scale research utilization project: "On the basis of the experience gained in this project, it is apparent that it was ahead of its proper time. When and if nursing research is identified, evaluated, and collated systematically, this project should be repeated on local levels in such a way that it is available to all nurses" [21].

Nursing Child Assessment Satellite Training (NCAST) Projects

Three projects were carried out between 1976 and 1985 with the purpose of translating and disseminating research findings. These projects aimed at increasing the practicing nurse's awareness of new research and the value of using research in practice. The first project (1976–1978) tested the use of a communications satellite for rapid dissemination of new research results that focused on new assessment techniques in child health. The second NCAST project (1978–1983) provided learners with videotaped parent-child interactions with which to practice assessments. The objective of the third NCAST project (1983–1985) was to teach public health nurses to use a nursing protocol for the follow-up care of preterm infants and their families [22].

Conduct and Utilization of Research in Nursing (CURN) Project

CURN, a five-year research development project, was funded by the Division of Nursing on the federal level from 1975 to 1980. The Michigan Nurses' Association conducted the project with the assistance of faculty and graduate students at the University of Michigan School of Nursing, the Institute for Social Research, and the Michigan State University School of Nursing. The purpose of the project was to improve the practice of nursing through two types of activities: (1) the utilization of existing research findings in the daily practice of registered nurses, and (2) the design and conduct of research that was directly relevant and could be readily transferred to nursing practice [23].

Thirty-four departments of nursing in hospitals throughout Michigan assisted the CURN project staff. The research utilization process developed and used by the project's staff consisted of a systematic series of activities that included: (1) the identification and synthesis of multiple-research studies in a common conceptual area (research base), (2) the transformation of the knowledge derived from a research base into a solution or clinical protocol, (3) the transformation of the clinical protocol into specific nursing actions (innovations) that are administered to patients, and (4) a clinical evaluation of the new practice to ascertain whether it produced the predicted result [24].

Ten research-based practice protocols were developed by CURN project personnel:

1. Preventing Decubitus Ulcers
2. Structured Preoperative Teaching
3. Clean Intermittent Catheterization
4. Intravenous Cannula Change
5. Reducing Diarrhea in Tube-Fed Patients
6. Closed Urinary Drainage Systems
7. Distress Reduction Through Sensory Preparation
8. Preoperative Sensory Preparation to Promote Recovery
9. Mutual Goal Setting in Patient Care
10. Pain: Deliberative Nursing Interventions

Each protocol was published as a separate book.* Horsley and colleagues (1981) provided a guide for implementation of the protocols. Each protocol in the series contains: (1) information regarding the need for the change (innovation); (2) a description of the innovation; (3) a summary of the research base provided by the conceptually related research studies that met

---

*See CURN Project. *Using Research to Improve Nursing Practice,* in the Bibliography and Suggested Readings section of this chapter.

specific criteria developed by CURN project personnel; (4) a description of research-based principles (empirical generalizations) guiding the implementation of the innovation; and (5) a description of the implementation and the systematic evaluation of its effects. Each protocol contains a summary of the benefits to be anticipated from successful use of the innovation, as well as additional pertinent materials.

In an effort to determine the extent of use of the CURN models in the practice setting, Brett used research journals and CURN publications to identify 14 nursing research findings that met the CURN project criteria for clinical use [25]. She then surveyed nurses practicing in small, medium, and large hospitals to determine the extent of their awareness of, persuasion about, and use of these research findings. All of the 216 respondents were full-time employees and were responsible for the direct care of patients; 86 percent were staff nurses and 14 percent were head nurses. Brett concluded: "The majority of nurses were aware of the average innovation, were persuaded about it, and use the average innovation at least sometimes." [26]. In a 1990 report of a replication of Brett's study, Coyle and Sokop found that, of the 113 nurses surveyed, the majority were aware of 9 of the 14 nursing practices and that 8 of the 14 practices were used regularly by more than half of the sample [27].

In 1987, Goode and her colleagues described how they used the CURN protocols to utilize research-based knowledge in their own hospital [28]. The already active audit committee was charged by the nursing administrator with reviewing, discussing, and evaluating findings from current research and making recommendations regarding the use of research findings in their hospital. The intent was to substantiate practice procedures with findings from current research. The authors provide three examples of completed research utilization projects. The first project they selected was temperature taking because not only did they want to start with an aspect of patient care to which all of their nurses could relate, but also there was concern about the basis for low temperature readings by the procedure currently in use. As a result of a review and evaluation of the research literature related to temperature taking, the committee found substantial support for making changes in hospital policies and procedures for temperature taking. They learned from this project that "Just because that is the way we've always done it is not reason enough to explain our practice" [29].

Subsequent utilization protocols were developed for preoperative teaching about coughing, deep breathing, and exercise and for a standardized teaching program on breast feeding. The nurses' use of research findings to drive their patient care decisions was an important contribution to positive patient outcomes. The authors concluded: "We are in our fifth year of work and the number of utilization projects is increasing. We hope this article encourages nurses to begin research utilization projects. There is nothing more rewarding than instituting a protocol based upon research that improves patient outcomes" [30].

The CURN protocols have continued to provide a model for developing research-based innovation protocols for nursing practice. These protocols represent a significant step in transferring research-based scientific knowledge into clinical nursing practice.

Research Utilization in the 1990s

In 1990, a significant advance in research utilization was made at the federal level with the creation of the Agency for Health Care Policy Research (AHCPR). This agency's primary goal is to enhance the quality, appropriateness, and effectiveness of health care services on a national basis. As one of its functions, it facilitates "the development, periodic review and updating of clinical practice guidelines . . . to assist practitioners in the prevention, diagnosis, treatment, and management of clinical conditions" [31]. Multidisciplinary panels comprised of physicians, nurses, and other experts conduct extensive literature searches related to the topic of the proposed guideline and then critically review and synthesize the literature to evaluate empirical evidence and significant outcomes. Panel recommendations are based primarily on published scientific literature; when the scientific literature is incomplete or inconsistent in a particular area, "the recommendations reflect the professional judgment of panel members and consultants" [32]. Among the practice guidelines developed by the AHCPR are guidelines on acute pain management (1992), urinary incontinence in adults (1992), prediction and prevention of pressure ulcers in adults (1992), and depression in primary care (1993). "For nurses wanting to base their practice on scientific evidence, these guidelines provide a basis for reviewing nursing policies, procedures, and protocols related to these . . . areas of care" [33].

Not only are the activities for utilization of research in nursing increasing, but there is no doubt that these activities will continue to be a major nursing focus well into the future. The current reality in the practice setting is that nurses must base their practice decisions on up-to-date scientific information. Standard VII of the American Nurses' Association (ANA) *Standards of Clinical Nursing Practice* states "the nurse uses research findings in practice" [34]. Nurses use interventions substantiated by research and participate in research activities "as appropriate to the individual's position, education, and practice environment." The nurse participates in research through such activities as critiquing research for application to practice and "using research findings in the development of policies, procedures, and guidelines for client care" [35]. The Joint Commission of the Association of Health Care Organizations (JCAHO) accreditation guidelines specify that patient care must be based on information from up-to-date sources about the design and performance of the process (such as practice guidelines). In addition, the commission specifies that the performance of this process must be compared to relevant scientific clinical and management literature. Not only are nuses being held increasingly accountable for current and scientifically based practice, but one writer asserts that "using research in practice represents a professional imperative. In fact, practice that does not incorporate up-to-date empirical findings may be unethical" [36].

The Research Utilization Process

Research utilization is a step-by-step process that facilitates movement from evaluating research studies to applying valid research findings in the practice setting. Just as you need to know the steps in the research process in order to evaluate a research study critically, you also need to know the basic steps in the research utilization process to be able to participate in utilization activities designed to apply research findings to clinical nursing practice. The following research utilization process incorporates much of the CURN model and that of the Horn model used by Goode and her colleagues [37].

1. Identify a clinical nursing problem to consider
2. Locate the research literature relevant to the clinical problem
3. Evaluate each research study critically for scientific merit and applicability to the clinical problem
4. Pool the critiques for each research study to determine if there is a sufficient research base, which is relevant to the clinical problem and could guide practice
5. If there is a sufficient research base, develop a research-based clinical protocol to address the clinical problem
6. Define the protocol's expected outcomes and formulate an evaluation plan
7. Educate personnel who will be involved in the use of the protocol
8. Do a trial run of the protocol on a pilot unit, evaluate the process and outcomes, and modify the protocol if indicated
9. Implement the protocol, evaluate, and revise as needed

The following example of the development of a research-based protocol for the management of asthma in school age children is provided to illustrate the application of the utilization process to a clinical nursing problem.

In identifying a clinical nursing problem, which could be improved if research findings were used, a group of elementary school nurses decided to establish a research-based intervention protocol to help asthmatic students and their families to manage asthma better. Because asthma is the number one chronic illness of childhood, school nurses frequently encounter these children in acute episodes and must be prepared to assess these students and refer them appropriately [38]. Because it is unwise to change practice based on the results of one study, the group then worked to locate multiple published research studies related to intervention for increasing coping and management skills of school age children with asthma. Since not all research reported in the literature is suitable for use in practice, the members critiqued each of the articles to determine the scientific merit and applicability to their clinical problem. They then pooled their critiques to determine if there was a sufficient research base that would be relevant to their clinical problem and that could guide the development of a management protocol for school nurses working with asthmatic children. The findings of their pooled critiques indicated that: (1) "instruction and support for asthmatic children is basic to the development of coping and management skills" and (2) school nurses are in a position to provide this instruction and support by organizing support groups within the school setting. These support groups would address such problems as the proper use of inhalers, the use of peak flow meters as objective measures of lung function, the proper pacing of activities, attention to the control of environmental factors for prevention, and self-help breathing and relaxation techniques [39].

After evaluating their pooled research findings for applicability to their clinical problem, the group decided there was a sufficient research base to develop a research-based clinical protocol. They then wrote a protocol for interventions that addressed "the issue of student coping and management skills designed to return the locus of control to the student and move toward reducing the frequency and severity of asthmatic episodes" [40]. This protocol incorporated what they determined to be the valid findings from their review of the research. Included in the protocol were management strategies during the acute phase of an asthmatic episode as well as long-term strategies that provided for students to participate in an asthma management support group. Their plan for implementing the asthma protocol in the school setting specified expected outcomes and proposed evaluation measures for both acute and long-term management. In order to educate the personnel who would be involved in using the protocol, they included plans for providing inservice education for all nurses who would be using the new protocol, as well as plans for the nurses to inservice school staff, counselors, and physical education teachers. They planned to conduct a trial run of the protocol in one school, evaluate the process and outcomes then modify the protocol if indicated.

These nurses addressed the management of children with asthma from the perspective of their own practice setting by using relevant research findings to develop a research-based protocol unique to their identified need. This is but one example of a range of research-based practice protocols that could be developed to guide practice in a specific setting.

Although a number of models for research utilization have been proposed in the literature, the approach identified in this chapter is intended to provide you with an understanding of the basic steps in research utilization. These basic steps can direct your participation in organizational activities designed to develop research-based protocols to guide clinical practice.

In summary, research utilization is concerned with using the results of scientific research to improve nursing practice. Systematic utilization of the results of valid research within organizational settings will ensure that patients receive scientifically based nursing care designed to enhance positive patient outcomes. It is crucial that nurses be prepared to participate in the research utilization process because they are being increasingly mandated to base their practice on scientific research. As a baccalaureate prepared nurse, you will need to be familiar with the research utilization process in order to participate in organizational activities to evaluate research critically, and to determine the readiness of the research for application to nursing practice as well as the design of research-based protocols. The activities in the Workbook will assist you to understand the process of deriving a research-based clinical protocol using the results of critical evaluation of research studies.

References

1. Horsley, J. A., J. Crane, M. Crabtree, and D. Wood. 1981. *Using Research to Improve Nursing Practice: A Guide.* New York: Grune and Stratton, pp. 1–2.
2. Horsley, J. 1985. "Using Research in Practice: The Current Context." *Western Journal of Nursing Research,* 7: 135.
3. Gennaro, S. 1994. "Research Utilization: An Overview." *JOGNN,* 4: 314.
4. Halpert, H. 1966. "Communications as a Basic Tool in Promoting Utilization of Research Findings." *Community Mental Health Journal,* 2 (Fall): 231.
5. Mercer, R. 1984. "Nursing Research: The Bridge to Excellence in Practice." *Image,* 16 (Spring): 47.

6. Burns, N., and S. K. Grove. 1993. *The Practice of Nursing Research: Conduct, Critique and Utilization,* 2nd ed. Philadelphia: Saunders, p. 668–669.

7. Diers, D. 1972. "Application of Research to Nursing Practice." *Image,* 5: 7–11.

8. Krueger, J., A. Nelson, and M. O. Wolanin. 1978. *Nursing Research: Development, Collaboration and Utilization.* Germantown, PA: Aspen Systems, p. 337.

9. Cronenwett, L. R. 1988. "Disseminating Research to Clinicians." *CNR,* 15: 1, 3.

10. Horsley et al. 1981. *Using Research to Improve Nursing Practice,* pp. xiii–xiv.

11. Ketefian, S. 1975. "Application of Selected Research Findings in Nursing Practice: A Pilot Study." *Nursing Research,* 24 (March–April): 91.

12. Kirchhoff, K. 1982. "A Diffusion Survey of Coronary Precautions." *Nursing Research,* 31 (July–August): 196–201.

13. Baessler, C. A., et al. 1994. "Medical-Surgical Nurses' Utilization of Research Methods and Products." *Medsurg Nursing,* 2: 120.

14. Kirchhoff, K. 1983. "Using Research in Practice: Should Staff Nurses Be Expected to Use Research?" *Western Journal of Nursing Research,* 5: 246.

15. Mercer, R. 1984. "Nursing Research: The Bridge to Excellence in Practice." *Image,* 16 (Spring): 47.

16. Hefferin, E., J. Horsley, and M. Ventura. 1982. "Promoting Research-Based Nursing: The Nurse Administrator's Role." *Journal of Nursing Administration,* May: 41.

17. Edwards-Beckett, J. 1990. "Nursing Research Utilization Techniques." *JONA,* 11: 25.

18. Lindeman, C., and J. Kreuger. 1977. "Increasing the Quality, Quantity, and the Use of Nursing Research." *Nursing Outlook,* 25 (July): 450.

19. Ibid., pp. 450–452.

20. Krueger, J., A. Nelson, and M. Wolanin. 1978. *Nursing Research: Development, Collaboration and Utilization.* Germantown, PA: Aspen Systems, p. 20.

21. Ibid., p. 337.

22. Crane, J. 1985. "Using Research in Practice: Research Utilization—Nursing Models." *Western Journal of Nursing Research,* 7: 494–497.

23. Krone, K., and M. Loomis. 1982. "Developing Practice-Related Research: A Model That Worked." *Journal of Nursing Administration,* April: 38.

24. Horsley et al. 1981. *Using Research to Improve Practice,* p. 2.

25. Brett, J. L. L. 1987. "Use of Nursing Practice Research Findings." *Nursing Research,* 36 (November–December): 344–349.
26. Ibid., p. 344.
27. Coyle, L. A., and A. G. Sokop. 1990. "Innovation Adoption Behavior Among Nurses." *Nursing Research,* 3: 176.
28. Goode, J. C., et al. 1987. "Use of Research Based Knowledge in Clinical Practice." *Journal of Nursing Administration,* 17 (December): 11–18.
29. Ibid., p. 13.
30. Ibid., p. 17.
31. Depression Guideline Panel. 1993. *Depression in Primary Care. Clinical Practice Guideline.* AHCPR Pub. 93-0550. Rockville, MD: Agency for Health Care Policy and Research, PHS, U.S. Department of Health and Human Services.
32. Ibid.
33. Mayhew, P. A. 1993. "Overcoming Barriers to Research Utilization with Research-Based Practice Guidelines." *Medsurg Nursing,* 4: 336.
34. American Nurses Association. 1991. *Standards of Clinical Nursing Practice.* Code No. NP 79 20M. Kansas City: American Nurses' Association, p. 16.
35. Ibid.
36. Mayhew, P. A. 1993. "The Importance of the Practicing Nurse in Nursing Research." *Medsurg Nursing,* 3: 211.
37. Horn Video Productions. 1991. *Research Utilization: A Study Guide.* Ida Grove, IA: Horn Video Productions, p. 26.
38. Peugh, S., et al. 1993. *Asthma Management for Elementary School Aged Children.* Paper presented at Sigma Theta Tau Regional Nursing Research Day. El Paso: TX, p. 1.
39. Ibid.
40. Ibid.

Bibliography and Suggested Readings

American Nurses Association. 1991. *Standards of Clinical Nursing Practice.* Kansas City: American Nurses Association.

Baessler, C. A., et al. 1994. "Medical-Surgical Nurses' Utilization of Research Methods and Products." *Medsurg Nursing,* 2: 113–121, 141.

Barnard, K. 1986. "Research Utilization: The Clinicians's Role." *MCN,* 3: 224.

Bostrom, J., and W. N. Suter. 1993. "Research Utilization: Making the Link to Practice." *Journal of Nursing Staff Development,* 1: 28–34.

Brett, J. L. 1987. "Use of Nursing Practice Research Findings." *Nursing Research,* 6: 344–349.

————. 1989. "Organizational Integrative Mechanisms and Adoption of Innovations by Nurses." *Nursing Research,* 2: 105–110.

Burns, N., and S. K. Grove. 1993. *The Practice of Nursing Research: Conduct, Critique, and Utilization,* 2nd ed. Philadelphia: W. B. Saunders.

Champion, V., and A. Leach. 1989. "Variables Related to Research Utilization in Nursing: An Empirical Investigation." *Journal of Advanced Nursing,* 14: 705–710.

Copp, L. 1990. "Research Dissemination Bottom Line and Bottom Drawer." *Journal of Professional Nursing,* 4: 187–188.

Coyle, L. A., and A. G. Sokop. 1990. "Innovation Adoption Behavior Among Nurses." *Nursing Research,* 3: 176–180.

Crane, J. 1985. "Using Research in Practice. Research Utilization: Theoretical Perspectives." *Western Journal of Nursing Research,* 7: 261–268.

Crane, J. 1985. "Using Research in Practice: Research Utilization—Nursing Models." *Western Journal of Nursing Research,* 7: 494–497.

Cronenwett, L. R. 1988. "Disseminating Research to Clinicians." *CRN,* 15: 3, 5.

CURN Project. *Using Research to Improve Nursing Practice.* New York: Grune and Stratton. Series of Clinical Protocols
Clean Intermittent Catheterization (1982)
Closed Urinary Drainage Systems (1981)
Distress Reduction through Sensory Preparation (1981)
Intravenous Cannula Change (1981)
Mutual Goal Setting in Patient Care (1982)
Pain: Deliberative Nursing Intervention (1982)
Preoperative Sensory Preparation to Promote Recovery (1981)
Preventing Decubitus Ulcers (1981)
Reducing Diarrhea in Tube-Fed Patients (1981)
Structured Preoperative Teaching (1981)

Depression Guideline Panel. 1993. *Depression in Primary Care. Clinical Practice Guideline.* AHCPR Pub. 93-0550. Rockville, MD: Agency for Health Care Policy and Research, PHS, U.S. Department of Health and Human Services.

Diers, D. 1972. "Application of Research to Nursing Practice." *Image,* 5: 7–11.

Dracup, K. A., and C. S. Breu. 1978. "Using Nursing Research Findings to Meet the Needs of Grieving Spouses." *Nursing Research,* 27 (July–August): 212–216.

Duffy, M. E. 1985. "Research Utilization: What's It All About?" *Nursing and Allied Health Care,* 6 (November): 474–475.

Edwards-Beckett, J. 1990. "Nursing Research Utilization Techniques." *JONA,* 11: 25–30.

Fawcett, J. 1984. "Another Look at the Utilization of Research. *Image,* 2: 59–62.

Friedman, M., and Z. Farag. 1991. "Gaps in the Dissemination/Knowledge Utilization Base." *Knowledge Creation Diffusion Utilization,* 3: 266–288.

Funk, S., E. Tornquist, and M. Champagne. 1989. "A Model for Improving the Dissemination of Nursing Research." *Western Journal of Nursing Research,* 3: 361–367.

———. 1989. "Application and Evaluation of the Dissemination Model." *Western Journal of Nursing Research,* 4: 486–491.

———. 1991. "Barriers to Using Research Findings in Practice: A Clinician's Perspective." *Applied Nursing Research,* 2: 90–95.

———. 1991. "Barriers: The Barriers to Research Utilization Scale." *Clinical Methods,* 1: 39–45.

Gennaro, Susan. 1994. "Research Utilization: An Overview. *JOGN,* 4: 313–319.

Goode, C. J., et al. 1987. "Use of Research Based Knowledge in Clinical Practice." *Journal of Nursing Administration,* 17 (December): 11–18.

Haller, K. B., M. A. Reynolds, and J. A. Horsley. 1979. "Developing Research-Based Innovation Protocols: Process, Criteria and Issues." *Research in Nursing and Health,* 2: 45–51.

Halpert, H. 1966. "Communications as a Basic Tool in Promoting Utilization of Research Findings." *Community Mental Health Journal,* 2 (Fall): 231.

Hefferin, E., J. Horsley, and M. Ventura. 1982. "Promoting Research-Based Nursing: The Nurse Administrator's Role." *Journal of Nursing Administration,* 12 (May): 34–41.

Horn Video Productions. 1991. *Research Utilization: A Study Guide.* Ida Grove, IA: Horn Video Productions.

Horsley, J. A. 1985. "Using Research in Practice: The Current Context." *Western Journal of Nursing Research,* 7: 135.

Horsley, J. A., J. Crane, and J. Bingle. 1978. "Research Utilization as an Organizational Process." *Journal of Nursing Administration,* 7: 4–6.

Horsley, J. A., et al. 1981. *Using Research to Improve Nursing Practice: A Guide.* New York: Grune and Stratton.

Hunt, M. 1987. "The Process of Translating Research Findings into Nursing Practice." *Journal of Advanced Nursing,* 12: 101–110.

Joint Commission of the Association of Health Care Organizations. 1994. *Accreditation Manual for Hospitals.* Oakbrook Terrace, IL: The Commission.

Ketefian, Shake. 1975. "Application of Selected Research Findings into Nursing Practice: A Pilot Study." *Nursing Research,* 24 (March–April): 89–92.

Kirchhoff, K. 1982. "A Diffusion Survey of Coronary Precautions." *Nursing Research,* 31 (July–August): 196–201.

———. 1983. "Using Research in Practice: Should Staff Nurses Be Expected to Use Research?" *Western Journal of Nursing Research,* 5: 246.

Krone, K., and M. Loomis. 1982. "Developing Practice-Related Research: A Model that Worked." *Journal of Nursing Administration,* 12 (April): 38.

Krueger, J. C., A. Nelson, and M. Wolanin. 1978. *Nursing Research: Development, Collaboration and Utilization.* Germantown, PA: Aspen Systems.

Lambert, C., and V. Lambert. 1988. "Clinical Nursing Research: Its Meaning to the Practicing Nurse." *Applied Nursing Research,* 2: 54–57.

Lindeman, C., and J. Krueger. 1977. "Increasing the Quality, Quantity, and the Use of Nursing Research." *Nursing Outlook,* 25 (July): 450.

———. 1984. "Dissemination of Nursing Research." *Image,* 16 (Spring): 57–58.

Longman, A., et al. 1990. "Research Utilization: An Evaluation and Critique of Research Related to Oral Temperature Measurement." *Applied Nursing Research,* 1: 14–19.

Loomis, M. 1985. "Knowledge Utilization and Research Utilization in Nursing." *Image,* 2: 35–39.

Marchette, L. 1985. "Developing a Productive Nursing Research Program in a Clinical Institution." *Journal of Nursing Administration,* 3: 25–29.

Mayhew, P. A. 1993. "The Importance of the Practicing Nurse in Nursing Research." *Medsurg Nursing,* 3: 210–211, 246.

Mayhew, P. A. 1993. "Overcoming Barriers to Research Utilization with Researched-Based Practice Guidelines." *Medsurg Nursing,* 4: 336–337.

Mercer, R. 1984. "Nursing Research: The Bridge to Excellence in Practice." *Image,* XVI, 47–51.

Peugh, S., et al. 1993. *Asthma Management for Elementary School Aged Children.* Paper presented at the Sigma Theta Tau Regional Nursing Research Day. El Paso, TX.

Stetler, C. 1985. "Research Utilization: Defining the Concept." *Image,* 2: 40–44.

Titler, M. G., et al. 1994. "Infusing Research Into Practice to Promote Quality Care." *Nursing Research,* 5: 307–313.

Tournquist, E., S. Funk, and M. Champagne. 1989. "Writing Research Reports for Clinical Audiences." *Western Journal of Nursing Research,* 5: 567–582.

Appendixes

The material in the appendix is designed to acquaint you with examples of different research proposals and guidelines for evaluating and preparing research reports and proposals. Appendixes A, B, and C provide you with examples of historical, quantitative, and qualitative research proposals. Appendix D outlines guidelines for evaluating a research report, while Appendix E provides guidelines for preparing a research proposal.

It is important to note that the research proposals in Appendixes A, B, and C have been reprinted to provide examples of a *format* for preparing a research proposal. Each proposal should be read with particular attention to the recommended format and style of a research proposal rather than for the currency of the material included in the proposal.

A Example of a Historical Research Proposal

ERNESTINE WIEDENBACH:
A HISTORICAL NURSING REVIEW
Her Life and Career Contributions
Susan Nickel*

Statement of the Problem
Literature Review
Conceptual Framework
Statement of the Purpose of the Study
Methodology
Plan for Data Analysis
Limitations of the Study

History makes the deeds of men (and women) live after them. Its function is to transmit knowledge of the past. It is a nation's memory, perpetuating its deeds, its traditions, and even its mistakes, also its aspirations and ideals. History makes the past a part of us, shapes our deeds in many ways, and links past and present with the future, making all one [1].

Statement of the Problem

Historical research deals with what has happened and how those happenings affect the present. More than a mere biography of a few leaders, historical research uses dates to determine the impact of events of the past on the present and occasionally tries to predict the future, based on this knowledge [2].

Historical research has long been a respected method of inquiry. A major contribution of historical inquiry is in the development of a broader, more complete perspective to enhance our understanding of the present and our approach to the future. Historical research is not merely a collection of incidents or facts; it is a study of the relationships of facts and incidents,

*Reprinted by permission of the author.

183

of themes or currents of social and professional issues that have influenced the present and the future [3].

Other professions, such as medicine, law, and education, have placed great importance on their histories and have used their knowledge of the past to guide and inspire their profession in its forward movement. The interest in historical nursing continues to lag. Some of the reasons for the dearth in nursing history include heavy teaching and administrative loads, salaries too meager to permit travel to archive sites, lack of local source material, and uncertainty of an outlet for publication [4]. Notter cited the lack of emphasis on nursing history taught in schools of nursing and the fact that nurses are too action-oriented as other possible causes.

> Research into present day problems without adequate search into the past to examine the course of events which produced the present problems, or bring to light past investigations of the same or similar problems by nurses or others, results in research which only scratches the surface and may even duplicate previous work. [5]

The role of historical research as a guide to the future becomes very clear as the lessons of the past are revealed. Provisions must be made so that nurses of the future may look back and draw both inspiration and direction from the nursing leaders of the past who have overcome obstacles. Ernestine Wiedenbach, B.A., M.A., R.N., P.H.N., C.N.M., has been a leader in the nursing profession since her graduation from the Johns Hopkins Hospital School of Nursing in 1925. Her five-decade career in nursing and nurse-midwifery has spanned a gamut of roles from practitioner to educator, administrator to author, patient advocate to mentor, and philosopher to theorist.

Today, Miss Wiedenbach lives in retirement in Miami, Florida. She is receptive and cooperative toward historical research on her life and career contributions. The value of her oral history of nursing and nurse-midwifery's past, present, and future as she perceives it is immeasurable.

Literature Review

Ernestine Wiedenbach's career has evolved continually through some difficult years for both nursing and our nation. She worked as a public health nurse during the Depression and with the American Nurses' Association/ National League for Nurses throughout World War II. When it was not widely accepted, she became a certified nurse-midwife. What prompted this woman from an upper-middle-class background to assume these various roles?

Role theory represents a collection of concepts and a variety of hypothetical formulations that predict how actors will perform in a given role, or under what circumstances certain types of behavior can be expected [6]. The body of scientific knowledge has grown markedly in recent years. Concomitantly, the field of health care has experienced a proliferation of roles. The exponential increase in technology in an extremely short time span and the demands made by consumers seeking ready access to care have caused health professionals to continually redefine and realign their roles. Nursing, like other professions, offers a career ladder for the aspiring. For career development, each upward step features different professional responsibilities, opportunities, and associations [7]. The shortage of primary care physicians created a situation in which clinical nurse specialists and nurse practitioners were hired to perform many clinical activities that were formerly the responsibility of physicians [8]. Brault, in a 1976 California study, found that nurses with higher levels of nursing responsibility were found to produce more favorable patient outcomes [9]. Clark and Affonso state:

> The number of roles which a person enacts also influences role performance ability. Someone with a repertoire of a variety of well practiced, realistic social roles is better able to meet new and critical situations and to deal effectively with others. However, a multiple of role demands may pose serious difficulties to a person's ability to fulfill role obligations unless the allocation of time and resources is handled in a satisfactory manner. [10]

Miss Wiedenbach has expressed her own concept of role theory: "Role may be conceptualized as a characterization of an individual of designated, distinctive qualities and competencies which (s)he typically manifests both in what (s)he does and in the way in which (s)he does it" [11]. She sees change in role as a behavioral response to the realities within the situation. Five realities noted in Miss Wiedenbach's role theory are: (1) the agent or propelling force, (2) the recipient or consumer, (3) the goal, (4) the means to the goal, and (5) the framework or environment. Role is expressed in any program of deliberate action, tempered by insight and the stock of resources [12]. To summarize, was Miss Wiedenbach's career development a product of the pressures of the health care settings and environment in which she worked, or was it a deliberately planned series of actions?

Conceptual Framework

The previously discussed role theory by Miss Wiedenbach will be used when analyzing data collected as it pertains to her career development. Also utilized as a background will be her central purpose to motivate the individual and/or facilitate her efforts to overcome the obstacles which currently or anticipatorily interfere with her ability to respond capably to the demands made of her by the realities in her immediate situation. [13]

Also as a framework will be the three fundamental concepts of her philosophy: (1) reverence for the gift of life; (2) respect for the dignity, worth, autonomy, and individuality of each human being; (3) resoluteness to act dynamically in relation to one's belief [14].

Statement of the Purpose of the Study

The purpose of this study is to contribute to the understanding of the history of nursing and nurse-midwifery by focusing on the life and career evolution of Ernestine Wiedenbach. The principal methodology will be oral history, recorded on video- and audiotapes. Interviews between the investigator and the research subject will be conducted in Miami, Florida.

A goal of the historiographer will be to establish the truth, publish the research findings, and establish a foundation for future historical research.

Methodology

The first step of this research study will be to gather background data, including a review of: (1) Miss Wiedenbach's writings; (2) the history of nursing in the United States, 1900 to 1970; (3) the birth and development of nurse-midwifery in the United States; and (4) a background history of the United States, 1900 to 1970.

Both primary and secondary source material will be used; however, the principal focus will be the valuable primary source of oral history as recorded from interviews with Ernestine Wiedenbach via audio and video tapings. Oral history is recognized as one of the most exciting current historical movements. The tapings of the remembrances of older members of a professional community provide records of what took place in the past periods of time and in specific places [15].

The profile of Miss Wiedenbach will focus on: personal data, personality characteristics, education, career evolution, philosophy, contributions, social relationships, reflections on nursing and nurse-midwifery, and predictions for the profession's future. Other primary sources used to substantiate the oral history will be published primary sources, personal writings, diaries, and professional societies' minutes and histories.

Secondary sources involve materials from some other authors. Although secondary sources are less reliable and trustworthy, they will be used as background material for corroboration. Particularly, information obtained from the Ernestine Wiedenbach Reading Room Archives at Yale University may provide interesting secondary sources. Review of these data may necessitate a trip to Yale by the researcher.

The historical research design will be used and all data will be subject to intensive internal and external criticism. External criticism establishes the validity of documents by examining the authenticity of the original material. The purpose of external criticism is to establish that original documents are what they purport to be. Examination of the handwriting, age of the paper, signature, and source are all part of the external criticism to prevent fraud.

Internal criticism establishes reliability of the data. An important part of internal criticism is a broad knowledge of the period in which the data originated. In this study, it would be important to bear in mind that even primary sources are not completely reliable and should be corroborated by two independent primary sources to be established as fact. Material will be categorized as a possibility when supported by only one primary source and a probability when supported by sufficient secondary source backing.

Thus, all information for this historical research must pass the criteria of internal and external criticism for reliability and validity.

Plan for Data Analysis

The narrative format will be used with synthesis of significant propositions. "The historian has no obligation to be clever or dull, but she had better be interesting" [16].

Limitations of the Study

Personal bias, projection of meaning, and incorrect interpretation of facts can pose a real problem to the historiographer. Objectivity must be maintained. Also considered as limitations will be the limited research experience of the investigator and time constraints.

References

1. Hockett, H. C. 1955. *Critical Method in Historical Research and Writing.* New York: Macmillan, p. 8.
2. Dempsey, P. A., and A. D. Dempsey. 1981. *The Research Process in Nursing.* New York: Van Nostrand, p. 117.
3. Notter, L. E. 1972. "The Case for Historical Research in Nursing." *Nursing Research,* 21 (November–December): 11.
4. Newton, M. E. 1965. "The Case for Historical Research." *Nursing Research,* 14 (Winter): 24.
5. Ibid., p. 23.

6. Hardy, M. E., and M. E. Conway. 1978. *Role Theory: Perspective for Health Professionals.* New York: Appleton-Century-Crofts, p. 24.
7. Ibid., p. 234.
8. Ibid., p. 179.
9. Ibid., p. 174.
10. Clark, A. L., and D. D. Affonso. 1976. *Childbearing: A Nursing Perspective.* Philadelphia: F. A. Davis, p. 50.
11. Wiedenbach, E. 1968. "The Nurse's Role in Family Planning." *Nursing Clinics of North America,* 3 (June): 356.
12. Ibid., p. 357.
13. Ibid., p. 358.
14. Ibid., p. 359.
15. Dempsey and Dempsey, *The Research Process,* p. 9.
16. Newton, "Historical Research," p. 23.

Bibliography

Baker, W. G. 1979. "Changes in Life Goals as Related to Success in a Nursing Leadership Role." *Nursing Research,* 28 (July–August): 234–236.

Christy, T. E. 1975. "The Methodology of Historical Research: A Brief Introduction." *Nursing Research,* 24 (May–June): 189–192.

Clark, A. L., and Affonso, D. D. 1976. *Childbearing: A Nursing Perspective.* Philadelphia: F. A. Davis.

Dempsey, P. A., and A. D. Dempsey. 1981. *The Research Process in Nursing.* New York: Van Nostrand.

Hardy, M. E., and M. E. Conway. 1978. *Role Theory: Perspectives for Health Professionals.* New York: Appleton-Century-Crofts.

Hockett, H. C. 1955. *Critical Method in Historical Research and Writing.* New York: Macmillan.

Newton, M. E. 1965. "The Case for Historical Research." *Nursing Research,* 14 (Winter): 20–26.

Notter, L. E. 1972. "The Case for Historical Research in Nursing." *Nursing Research,* 21 (November–December): 11–12.

Varney, H. 1980. *Nurse-Midwifery.* Boston: Blackwell Scientific.

Wiedenbach, E. 1968. "The Nurse's Role in Family Planning." *Nursing Clinics of North America,* 3 (June): 355–365.

B Example of a Quantitative Proposal

COMPLIANCE WITH UNIVERSAL PRECAUTIONS
IN PEDIATRIC SETTINGS
*Jacqueline C. Williams**

> **Introduction and Statement of the Problem**
> **Literature Review**
> **Conceptual Framework**
> **Purpose of the Study**
> **Definition of Terms**
> **Plan for Data Collection**
> **Plan for Data Analysis**
>   Sample Data Table
> **Limitations of the Study**

Introduction and Statement of the Problem

Bloodborne pathogens, particularly human immunodeficiency virus (HIV) and Hepatitis B (HBV) have been identified as significant threats to health care workers [1]. To counter this threat consistently, the Occupational Safety and Health Administration (OSHA) issued definitive guidelines on Universal Precautions (UP), delineating the responsibilities of both the employer and health care worker in avoiding exposure to body fluids, which could serve as a vector for transmission of diseases [2, 3]. Employers were mandated to provide two critical elements: (1) education of employees in the use of UP, and (2) provision of the protective equipment needed to implement the system (i.e., gloves, gowns, eye goggles, and puncture-proof containers for sharp objects).

Health care workers, however, have frequently failed to comply consistently with UP guidelines [4]. Nurses have figured prominently in the concern about this phenomenon since nurses constitute the largest single group of health care workers who have experienced seroconversion to HIV [1]. Studies conducted in specialized and general areas of clinical practice

*Reprinted by permission of the author.

have yielded similar results and identified various reasons for noncompliance with UP.

After several years of involvement with teaching UP in and out of the hospital setting, the researcher became interested in observing nurses involved with pediatric patients, focusing in particular on the decreased attention to UP that is exhibited when nurses work with children in a general hospital setting. Informal inquiry into this observation indicated that the nurses were often sacrificing the safety of UP in an effort to increase efficiency because of their anxiety and desire to do procedures, such as venipuncture, as expediently as possible.

Although some studies have focused on practice areas where children may be seen (e.g., emergency room, surgery), there is little data found in the literature that specifically applies to pediatric practice settings. Neither are there studies on how the special problems of pediatric practice may influence risk-taking by nurses in this regard; in light of the fact that the threat of pathogens continues to expand in all populations [5], re-evaluation of compliance rates as an important facet of monitoring the effectiveness of employee education about UP is important to nursing administration, infection control, employee health, and education departments. The questions posed for this study are: What are the rates of compliance to UP by registered nurses working with pediatric populations in hospital settings, and how are the age of the children, and the size and type of hospital related to compliance?

Literature Review

The concept of UP was formalized on recommendations of the CDC and OSHA [6]. UP represents the minimal actions that can be taken by employers and health care workers to avoid exposure to bloodborne pathogens [1]. These precautions become more important as the number of HIV and HBV-infected patients continues to increase [7]. Compliance with UP, assuming that health care workers have knowledge of the system and are equipped with an adequate supply and quality of barrier equipment, is the responsibility of the individual.

Many studies in the past 5 years reveal that health care workers, including nurses, fail to follow UP [4]. Studies can be grouped into two types: (1) those reporting on overall compliance rates and (2) those focusing on specific portions of UP (glove use, for example). Gauthier et al. noted only one study on compliance rates in which more than two of the four aspects of UP protocols (barrier precautions, hand washing, handling of sharp instruments, and avoidance of unprotected mouth-to-mouth resuscitation) were assessed simultaneously [4]. Basically, two types of tools have been used by researchers to judge compliance rates: direct observation and retrospective, written surveys.

Kelen used direct observation in an emergency room setting and scored overall compliance with UP as 44 percent, reporting the observed staff did not use appropriate precautions with 2275 patients whose HIV status was unknown [8]. Another observational study reviewed by McNabb and Keller was conducted in 1987 by Gerberding and colleagues at San Francisco General Hospital where 56 percent of health care workers took inadequate precautions even when dealing with known AIDS patients [9, 10]. Becker and coworkers gathered data on recapping of needles, significant in that needle-stick exposure to bloodborne pathogens is currently the source of most serious exposure [11]. They counted uncapped needles in disposal boxes in the four largest hospitals in southeast Michigan where 75 percent of the state's AIDS patients were admitted. Even after intensive campaigns to change the habit of capping needles, three of the four hospitals found needle recapping rates of 25 percent to 50 percent. The Center for Devices and Radiologic Health, collaborating with some state health departments in conducting an observation, found that glove usage was substantial but not universal [12]. Observational studies of hand washing demonstrated doctors and nurses failed to wash their hands after patient contact 59 percent of the time [9].

Studies using retrospective, written survey methods were more common. Stotka and colleagues delineated the frequency of exposure by all types of health care workers on acute-care medical wards at two large hospitals in Virginia, finding that blood exposure to hands during intravenous procedures and manipulations and blood glucose tests was the most common problem [7]. In 75 percent of the exposures, failure to use a barrier device, usually gloves, was noted. McNabb and Keller conducted an in-depth survey of nurses and risk-taking in regard to HIV transmission [9]. Despite the fact they found that nurses had adequate knowledge and beliefs about HIV and UP protocols, 76 percent of the respondents reported at least one unprotected exposure to blood and body fluids in the week preceding their completion of the questionnaire [9].

In another study, Wiley, Heath, Acklin, Earl, and Barnard found that 20 percent, 64 out of the 323 nurses surveyed, believed they had been exposed, through mucous membranes or broken skin, to blood and body fluids of an HIV-positive patient [13]. The hospital employee health records of this medical center had only seven such reports on file, indicating that many exposures may go unreported. This applied to other aspects of exposure as various studies indicate needle sticks are unreported as much as 53 percent of the time and that 57 percent of the hands of health care workers examined in the study conducted by Saghafi and colleagues had acute or chronic lesions, which would make skin contact with body fluids dangerous [9, 14]. Burtis and Evangelisti noted that 40 to 60 percent of nurses surveyed at their institutions used UP inappropriately in caring for known AIDS patients by the *over-cautious* use of double gloving or *overuse* of other

barrier precautions [15]. The international nature of the problem is illustrated by the fact that articles on problems with UP compliance were available from countries other than the United States [14, 16].

The purposes for which studies on UP compliance are conducted, reveal
the complexity of the problem. Many studies tried to identify how knowledge levels were related to behaviors [5, 9, 13, 15, 17]. The studies represent results of "educating" nurses into compliance. A second type of study
aimed at identification of situations where exposure most often occurs so
that education, institutional policy, and the provision of supplies could be
altered to counter the threat [7, 9, 17].

Throughout the literature review there was widespread consensus that
nurses generally have the knowledge to understand UP compliance and
are choosing not to do so for a variety of poorly understood reasons. This
is not a static problem. As new efforts to improve compliance are tested,
ongoing evaluation is needed.

Conceptual Framework

In viewing the issue of nurses' compliance with UP, it is obvious that the
problem has far-reaching implications. Institutional compliance with
OSHA requirements has not been matched by compliance rates from individuals. King's open systems framework and its resultant theory of goal
attainment are chosen for this study as a systematic way to analyze and
evaluate UP compliance.

The open systems framework is a model envisioning all human relations,
including nursing, as occurring within three interacting systems: personal,
interpersonal, and social [18]. Certain key concepts occur in each of these
systems as represented here.

Key Concepts in King's Interacting Systems Framework

Personal System	Interpersonal System	Social System
Perception	Interaction	Organization
Self	Communication	Authority
Growth and development	Transaction	Power
Body image	Role	Status
Space	Stress	Decision making
Time	Coping	

The personal system includes perception, self, growth and development,
body image, space, and time. The interpersonal system includes interaction, communication, transaction, role, stress, and coping. A social system

contains the social roles, the practices and the behaviors that are developed to maintain values; these include organization, authority, power, status, and decision making. By extension, knowledge of UP protocols resides within the personal system of the individual nurse, usage in a patient care situation occurs on an interpersonal level, and accountability for compliance is a function of the social systems, such as a hospital, or more globally, the federal government through OSHA regulations.

King's application of the interacting systems model is represented by the goal attainment theory [18, 19]. The overall goal of nursing is to assist individuals to maintain a state of health. Many of the problems revolving around the issues of bloodborne pathogens can be viewed more clearly in this context. If it were possible for patients and nurses to know one another's HIV status for example, bloodborne pathogens could be treated the same as other forms of contagion. But the peculiarities of the infection and the requirement of confidentiality make reliable identification of carriers of the infections impossible. The nurse's inability to *perceive* which individuals represent true risks is because this vital bit of knowledge cannot be *communicated* between the nurse and patient in most situations. The concept of UP has been chosen to replace that knowledge. Operating on the assumption that any client or any care giver could be carrying a bloodborne disease, UP is utilized in all physical *transactions,* whether disease is actually present or not, to attain the goal of preventing transmission of the bloodborne disease.

Within the social system of a health care institution, the employer has a mandated ethical and fiscal responsibility to both clients and employees as a result of legal precedents and such global social agencies as OSHA. The hospital *perceives* the nurse to be at risk for exposure to bloodborne pathogens, *communicates* expectations, encourages feedback and information, provides resources, and oversees the mutual expectation of guarding the nurse and client alike against exposure.

This research proposal represents only a small segment of the complicated processes of monitoring UP compliance. It is an attempt to document how well nurses are complying with UP in a specific setting with a subset of the population in the social system of hospitals in the Southwestern part of the United States. The information obtained from this study can be evaluated with the open systems framework, and that system can be used to suggest areas for further evaluation or action.

The subject of motivating nurses to follow UP guidelines may be analyzed in better perspective when viewed within the interacting systems framework. For example, nurses indicated a need for institutions to get more input from them in making and carrying out policies in regard to many aspects of bloodborne disease policies and procedures [9, 13, 15]. Viewed in the open systems framework, this represents a failure in the interpersonal realm of *communication,* which may result in the social system *making decisions* that are not suited for attaining the goal of providing the means and incentive for nurses to avoid exposure to bloodborne pathogens. Researchers also noted that knowledge alone was a poor predictor of compliance to UP [9, 11, 17]. "Reminder" campaigns were found to have transitory, rather than permanent, effects on compliance [9, 11]. Other studies indicated that situational factors have a great influence on compliance rates and that mandated compliance policies may be more productive in achieving the goal of increased compliance than general knowledge [9, 17].

Purpose of the Study

The purpose of this study is to describe the rates of compliance to UP by registered nurses working with pediatric populations in hospital settings and to analyze how the age of the child may have an impact on compliance. It is important to know if some of the special challenges of working with pediatric age groups (such as difficult IV starts, the high acuity of hospitalized children, and so on) will be reflected in compliance rates. There is little published data on the trends for the southwestern United States, therefore this study can add to the body of knowledge concerning UP protocols.

Definition of Terms

To prevent confusion of terminology the following definitions will be used:

Universal Precautions (UP)   a system approved by the Center for Disease Control that includes avoidance of exposure to blood and body fluids that can harbor Hepatitis B and human immunodeficiency viruses. Fluids that always require UP are blood, semen, vaginal secretions, cerebral spinal, pleural, peritoneal, pericardial, synovial and amniotic fluids. Fluids of mucous membranes are considered to require UP.

Compliance   appropriate use of barrier equipment, handwashing, disposal of sharps, and resuscitation and ventilation devices to avoid a nurse's exposure to blood or body fluids of clients as outlined by UP.

Opportunity for compliance   any action or interaction of the nurse in a client care situation, which could result in an exposure and during which UP should be used as judged by a trained observer.

Exposure   transfer of blood or any of the body fluids listed under the definition for UP, into the bloodstream, onto mucous membranes, or onto the nonintact skin of a nurse.

Pediatric patient   a client age 18 years or younger.

General hospital   one treating a wide range of ages and conditions and including pediatric services with at least one medical/surgical inpatient unit.

Pediatric hospital   hospital in which all clients fall into the pediatric population.

Plan for Data Collection

This study is a descriptive study of registered nurses at medium and large general and pediatric hospitals in the southwestern United States. It will include one or more pediatric medical/surgical units in each of four hospitals. Medical/surgical units are included due to the relatively high acuity seen there and because they can be found in both large and small hospitals. Two of the hospitals will be general hospitals with pediatric services and two will be pediatric hospitals. One general and one pediatric hospital will be approximately 250 beds, while the other general hospital and pediatric hospital will be greater than 500 beds.

The target population will be all registered nurses on pediatric medical/surgical units observed in their practice setting with pediatric clients in the four different hospitals selected for the study. The sample will consist of 30 registered nurses from each of the 4 hospitals and will be chosen by using a random numbers table where staffs are large enough to make observing all of them prohibitive.

The research team will include a project coordinator and individuals identified by the infection control departments of the four hospitals in the study who will be trained to collect the observational data.

An adapted version of The Universal Precautions Assessment Tool (UPAT) devised by Dorothy Gauthier and colleagues at the University of Alabama at Birmingham School of Nursing will be used to collect the data [4]. The tool is designed to collect data related to compliance to the four major components of UP: handwashing, barrier precautions, disposal of sharps, and use of resuscitation/ventilation devices. It is a one-page tool on which an observer records whether the proper procedure is followed by the nurse by marking the corresponding *yes* or *no* space on the checklist. The individual's score is obtained as a percentage of correct responses per number of opportunities noted for complying with UP while working with patients. A separate section records demographic data and will be modified from the original tool to add the age of the child (in months) in addition to the hospital unit, observation times, nurse code, observer initials, and final score. One score sheet per child will be used. Two observers will simultaneously score the same nurse caring for a child.

The UPAT can be used to assess compliance individually and collectively. The authors of the tool established its consensual validity by submitting it for review to three experts in infection control during their two pilot studies [4]. It is described as being able to analyze, by category, the strengths and weaknesses of personnel in compliance with UP. The data can be further compared for these variables by adding space for the age of patient and category of hospital. Anonymity of both the nurse and patient will be preserved by using only codes on the score sheets.

Observers will be trained in the use of the instrument by the researcher. The original authors conducted tests of interrater reliability in two pilot tests by having observers simultaneously rate the same nurses and using an intraclass correlation coefficient to compare the scoring. The tool was found to have an interrater reliability score within the 95 percent confidence limits [4]. Interrater reliability scores will be calculated in the same way for this study.

Observers will spend 45 to 60 minutes either continuously or intermittently observing each of the study subjects during the nurses' regular shifts. To accustom the staff to the presence of the observers, members of the research team will spend some time on the unit in other infection control activities prior to beginning use of the UPAT. Because the hospitals have an obligation to monitor compliance to UP throughout their facility, individual informed consent will not be obtained. Gauthier and colleagues tested this instrument under these conditions by informing subjects prior to observations that the observers were noting either patient care or nursing activities and that the results were to be used in a study.

Plan for Data Analysis

The UPAT will yield a series of compliance scores. Since there is an ideal individual level of compliance with UP (100%), the compliance scores for each subject will be expressed as percentages (e.g., nurse was observed to comply with UP 75% of the time). UPAT will provide a score for each major category of UP (handwashing, use of barrier precautions, handling of sharps, and use of resuscitation/ventilation devices), as well as an overall score. The raw scores will be used in the statistical analysis. The chi squared (χ^2) statistic will be used to determine if there are statistically significant differences in nurses' compliance with UP based on hospital setting and age of the child. The UPAT will also allow a comparison of compliance rates within the categories of UP itself. For example, handwashing use can be analyzed separately from the other three elements of UP.

Sample Data Table

The following is a cross-comparison of compliance scores for all nurses in the study by UP categories and the age of the child (in months).

UP Categories	Age of Child (months)				
	0–12	13–36	37–72	73–144	145–216
Barrier precautions					
Hand washing					
Disposal of sharps					
Resuscitation/ventilation devices					

Limitations of the Study

The UPAT is a relatively new tool that has both advantages and limitations. One strength is its concise assessment of all the categories of UP. It avoids the bias of self-reporting tools, which have been associated with significant under-reporting due to lack of awareness and poor recall over a period of time [9, 14].

This study has several limitations. The most significant is the Hawthorne effect as all subjects will be aware they are being observed. Having members of the research team come from within the hospital and spend some preliminary time on the target unit can lessen, but not eliminate this effect. Another limitation is that scoring will rely on the judgment of the observer. For example, CDC guidelines advise glove usage for phlebotomy when the *phlebotomist* perceives a risk to blood exposure to be probable. The authors of the UPAT suggest research teams will need to confer during the training phase to agree on ground rules for such situations to control for this possibility. A final limitation is that grouping the data for the proposed analyses (such as age group comparisons) may result in decreased cell sizes necessary for statistical testing and may affect determination of statistical significance.

References

1. Centers for Disease Control. 1988. Update: Universal Precautions for Prevention of Transmission of Human Immunodeficiency Virus, Hepatitis B Virus, and other Bloodborne Pathogens in Health Care Settings. *MMWR,* 37: 377–382.
2. Department of Labor. 1987. Joint Advisory Notice, Department of Labor. Department of Health and Human Services. HBV HIV. *Federal Register,* 52: 41818–41823.
3. Department of Labor. 1989. Occupational Safety and Health Administration. Occupational Exposure to Bloodborne Pathogens: Proposed Rule and Notice of Hearing. *Federal Register,* 54: 23134–23139.
4. Gauthier, D. K., et al. 1991. "Monitoring Universal Precautions: A New

Assessment Tool." *Infection Control and Hospital Epidemiology,* 12: 597–601.

5. Huerta, S. R., and Oddi, L. R. 1992. "Refusal to Care for Patients with Human Immunodeficiency/Acquired Immunodeficiency Syndrome: Issues and Responses." *Journal of Professional Nursing,* 8: 221–230.

6. Miramontes, H. 1990. "Progress in Establishing Safety Protocols Based on CDC and OSHA Recommendations." *Infection Control and Hospital Epidemiology* (supplement), 11: 561–562.

7. Stotka, J. L., et al. 1991. "An Analysis of Blood and Body Fluid Exposures Sustained by House Officers, Medical Students, and Nursing Personnel on Acute-care General Medical Wards: A Prospective Study." *Infection Control and Hospital Epidemiology,* 12: 583–590.

8. Kelen, G. D., et al. 1989. "Human Immunodeficiency Virus Infection in Emergency Department Patients: Epidemiology, Clinical Presentations and Risk to Health Care Workers—The Johns Hopkins Experience." *JAMA* 262: 516–522.

9. McNabb, K., and Keller, M. L. 1991. "Nurses' Risk Taking Regarding HIV Transmission in the Workplace." *Western Journal of Nursing Research,* 13: 732–745.

10. Gerberding, J. L., et al. 1987. "Risk of Transmitting Human Immunodeficiency Virus, Cytomegalovirus, and Hepatitis B to Health Care Workers Exposed to Patients with AIDS and AIDS-Related Conditions." *Journal of Infectious Diseases,* 156: 1–7.

11. Becker, M. H., et al. 1990. "Noncompliance with Universal Precautions Policy: Why do Physicians and Nurses Recap Needles?" *American Journal of Nursing,* 18: 232–239.

12. Kaczmarek, R. G., et al. 1991. "Glove Use by Health Care Workers: Result of a Tristate Investigation." *American Journal of Infection Control,* 19: 228–232.

13. Wiley, K., et al. 1990. "Care of HIV-infected Patients: Nurses' Concerns, Opinions, and Precautions." *Applied Nursing Research,* 3: 27–33.

14. Saghafi, L., et al. 1992. "Exposure to Blood during Various Procedures: Results of Two Surveys Before and After the Implementation of Universal Precautions." *American Journal of Infection Control,* 20: 53–57.

15. Burtis, R. E., and Evangelisti, J. T. 1992. " 'Will Universal Precautions Protect Me?' A Look at Staff Nurses' Attitudes." *Nursing Outlook,* 40: 133–138.

16. Wills, D. J. 1990. "Inadvertent Occupational Exposure to Blood and Adherence to Universal Precautions: Pilot Study." *New Zealand Nursing Forum,* 18: 7–9.

17. Gruber, M., et al. 1989. "The Relationship Between Knowledge about Acquired Immunodeficiency Syndrome and Implementation of Univer-

sal Precautions by Registered Nurses." *Clinical Nurse Specialist,* 3: 182–185.

18. King, I. 1981. *A Theory for Nursing: Systems, Concepts, Process.* New York: J. Wiley.

19. Fawcett, J. 1989. "King's Interacting Systems Framework." In *Analysis and Evaluation of Conceptual Models of Nursing.* Philadelphia: F. A. Davis Company, pp. 99–129.

C   Example of a Qualitative Research Proposal

HOMELESS PERSONS WITH AIDS LIVING IN A CONGREGATE FACILITY: AN ETHNOGRAPHIC STUDY
*Suzan Jaffe**

> **Introduction and Statement of the Problem**
> **Literature Review**
> **Purpose of the Study**
> **Plan for Data Collection**
> Study Design
> Setting
> Sample
> Data Collection Techniques
> **Plan for Data Analysis**
> **Limitations of the Study**
> **Ethical Considerations**
> **Nursing Implications**
> **Appendix A: Interview Schedule**
> **Appendix B: Informed Consent Form—**
> **Living in Sunrise Manor**

Introduction and Statement of the Problem

Acquired immunodeficiency syndrome (AIDS) is now the leading cause of death in the United States in men under 45 years of age. It is reported that over 100,000 persons in the United States have been diagnosed as having AIDS. Nearly half of these persons with AIDS (PWAs) have died (Center for Disease Control, 1989).

Most PWAs are not hospitalized until an AIDS-related infection with serious physical or psychological debilitation necessitates admission. As such, most PWAs live at home, alone, with friends or family. The financial

The author of this appendix wishes to thank Dr. Lydia DeSantis for her professional guidance and editorial assistance in preparing this proposal.
*Reprinted by permission of the author.

burden to PWAs is often unmanageable. It can be devastating to someone who prior to diagnosis had inadequate insurance coverage. For PWAs without insurance or family support, the ramifications of having AIDS are overwhelming and can result in one's becoming homeless.

At present there exist but a few shelters or congregate living facilities in the United States that offer food and shelter for homeless PWAs. Having AIDS is saturated with its own unique set of physical, psychological, and social puzzles. Being homeless is accompanied by a multitude of problems. Being a homeless PWA is a contemporary condition, and the needs of this group have not been clearly identified.

There are over 4 million homeless in the United States. According to a published study, the typical homeless person in South Florida has a high school education, a family to support, a drug and alcohol problem or both, and nowhere to turn for help. In Dade, Broward, and Palm Beach counties there are about 17,000 individuals who, despite their "homelessness," do not fit the stereotypical "skid row" street bums. Fifty percent are families headed by single women. Fifty-five percent suffer from untreated psychiatric illnesses. Approximately 30 percent have untreated drug and alcohol addictions. It is estimated that 11 percent of the homeless in Miami alone have AIDS (Dewar, 1989).

Despite the apparent interest and the abundance of published information on and about PWAs and homelessness, the literature has focused on the person either caring for PWAs or on those persons living with PWAs. Literature describing what it is like to be a homeless PWA from the PWA's perspective is lacking, but is a necessary first step in addressing the needs and planning appropriate interventions for this growing population.

Literature Review

The literature considers HIV-infected (human immunodeficiency virus infected) individuals from a multiplicity of ethnic cultures and subcultures within these ethnic groups. Even though issues pertaining to specific cultural groups are mentioned, the predominant discussion and source of knowledge is not from an emic perspective (that of the participant). For example, what it is like to live in the United States as an African-American male IV drug user may change dramatically once this individual becomes infected with HIV or is labeled as having AIDS. The cultural rules and expected behaviors may be significantly transformed. How this individual perceives his world may also be modified.

In an investigation by Kelly et al. (1987), physicians' attitudes toward AIDS patients were explored. Kelly concluded that one of the strongest attitudes was that PWAs are responsible for their illness. In an ethnographic study, Denker (1986) examined the perspectives of health care workers toward pediatric AIDS patients in a large metropolitan city hospital. Seven major themes or domains emerged from this study. These included (1) care, (2) knowledge regarding AIDS, (3) geography within the patient care unit, (4) infection control, (5) fears and doubts, (6) growth and development, and (7) beliefs, feelings, and emotional responses. Denker concluded that most of the fears concerning caring for the pediatric AIDS patients were based on "unknowns"—fears rooted in the uncertainties of viral spread. Education and on-the-job experience with pediatric AIDS patients were the most important factors in decreasing health care workers' unfounded fears.

Freidson (1974) noted that individuals with sexually transmitted diseases were often held in lower respect by medical professionals. The attitude of health care workers has reinforced the stigma of AIDS, with the result that high-risk groups (regardless of their seropositivity status) are even further feared by society. If an illness is discredited by the medical (professional) community, there appears to be more likelihood of stigmatization of the affected persons.

Almost all aspects of AIDS can be considered a social phenomenon. The characterization of high-risk individuals as being primarily the homosexual and drug addict groups made AIDS a stigmatized disease almost immediately. The uncertainties of AIDS are endless, and being labeled as an HIV-infected individual or a PWA may be an obstacle to social interaction, employment, and insurance qualification. As such, the positive characteristics of an individual may be ignored.

Not since the plagues of the sixteenth century and the views of syphilis during the seventeenth century has a disease earned so much social consequence. The social response to AIDS has been such that even highly educated health care professionals interpret the disease as a punishment for social and sexual deviance (Kelly et al., 1987).

In twentieth-century America, AIDS has clearly been related to certain types of antisocial behavior. Fear generated by the uncertainties of AIDS is a common emotional response of all groups (Cassens, 1985). As recently as 1986, children with AIDS made headlines and were banned from attending public school. Headlines such as "Gay plague, lethal scourge, and mysterious epidemic" (McCombie, 1986, p. 457) have fashioned AIDS into a highly stigmatized disease. Persons infected with HIV, as well as suspected (by the public) of infection, have been openly shunned and alienated. The media have often referred to the blameless innocent victims (children and hemophiliacs) being infected by the guilty (homosexuals and IV drug abusers).

In Goffman's (1963) classic work, *stigma* was defined as an attribute, an undesired differentness, that discredits or disqualifies the individual from full social acceptance. This "differentness" was not in itself cause for social disqualification, but rested on an interactional process through which this differentness was given social significance and meaning. It was the public's reaction, therefore, that measured the inner strength of a social norm (Shoham and Rahav, 1970).

Some diseases are clearly more biophysically discrete or recognizable. Venereal diseases have been associated with clandestine or immoral sexual activities. Freidson (1974) states that in certain cases, such as venereal disease, there is a moralistic judgment of blame and the indisposed is held responsible for the diseased state. The concept of stigma as some type of repercussion of norm violation is almost universal. The interpretation of such marks or signs is culturally defined, and the position of the one doing the stigmatizing is influential.

Research reports and articles in the medical, nursing, and behavioral sciences are saturated with articles about AIDS, its etiology and pathogenesis; its impact on sexual behaviors and practices, drug addiction, health care delivery, employment, and discrimination issues (Kelly et al., 1987). These reports, however, have only minimally addressed the perspectives and attitudes of PWAs.

Purpose of the Study

The purpose of this study is to describe what it is like to be a homeless PWA living in a congregate facility.

Plan for Data Collection

Study Design

A naturalistic inquiry using ethnographic methodology will be the approach used to conduct this investigation. Ethnography is a method by which a culture or subculture can be described. The final product of the ethnographic method is a written report based on the description and analysis of the culture of concern.

Ethnography has been defined in the nursing literature as the systematic process of observing, detailing, describing, documenting, and analyzing the lifeways or particular patterns of a culture (or subculture) (Leininger, 1985). Ethnographic methodology is an ideal way to identify behaviors and generate knowledge that will establish the groundwork for further research. Homeless PWAs living in a congregate facility can be considered a subculture whose life-ways are as yet unidentified. The ethnographic approach provides the most appropriate means for describing what living in the congregate setting is like from the perspective of PWAs.

Setting

A church-affiliated congregate living facility opened in 1988 in South Florida. It accepts PWAs who have nowhere else to go and who otherwise would probably be forced to live on the streets. All persons living in this setting have a diagnosis of AIDS or have had an AIDS-related infection or complication. This congregate residence has been selected as the field setting for the researcher's ethnographic study. For anonymity, this residence will be given the fictional name "Sunrise Manor."

Sample

The sample for this study will be drawn from those PWAs living full time at Sunrise Manor. The sampling approach will be a purposive sample of convenience. Residents' charts, containing medical, family, and social histories, will be available for the investigator's review. To avoid preconceived views toward residents and the risk of biasing sample selection, the investigator will not review the charts until after the participants have been selected.

Four to six residents (male and female) will be interviewed in a series of in-depth interviews. It is also anticipated that the staff will be observed as they interact with the residents and will be spoken with informally. It is contemplated that the investigator will spend 15 to 30 hours a week in the field setting.

Data Collection Techniques

Data will be obtained primarily by observation and participant observation. Participant observation will combine straight observation and both unstructured and structured interviews. An interview schedule will be developed before each formal interview. After analysis of each interview, new questions will be generated and, if possible, follow-up interviews will be scheduled. Questions will be of the grand-tour and mini-tour variety (as discussed in Spradley, 1979). An example of the initial interview schedule is attached (Appendix A).

A tape recorder will be used whenever possible during formal and informal interviews. Once transcribed, the tapes will be kept for review in order to listen to the residents' articulation and exclamation and to facilitate a further appreciation of their moods. At the completion of this study, the tapes will be erased.

Because the investigator anticipates the use of photography as adding an important dimension to the data base and as facilitating content analysis, a camera will be used (when permitted and appropriate) to capture germane scenes. Photographs allow the researcher to witness an event, situation, or condition through the camera and simultaneously to become a participant observer. This is accomplished by using the camera as an instrument or tool of social inquiry and education. All photographs, including negatives, will be destroyed upon completion of the study. In addition to photographs, hand-drawn sketches, and maps and floor plans of the living quarters and private and public areas of Sunrise Manor will be interpreted throughout the data presentation process to better orient the reader to the setting.

Plan for Data Analysis

According to Lincoln and Guba (1985), within the ethnographic paradigm, data analysis is not a matter of reduction but of induction. Inductive analysis begins with the data analysis, rather than from established theories or hypotheses. The investigator will use the transcriptions of the interviews and field notes as the source of data analysis. Words and word combinations will be selected so that the researcher can identify the significant area for analysis. Recurrent combinations will generate conceptualizations, understandings, and trends from the perspective of PWAs living in Sunrise Manor.

Limitations of the Study

Since the sample will be drawn from a group of homeless PWAs living in a specific setting, the conclusions cannot be generalized to all PWAs living in congregate facilities, or to all homeless.

Ethical Considerations

The protocol for this research study, initial interview schedule, and informed consents will be submitted to the appropriate institutional review boards responsible for the protection of human subjects involved in research. Three different consent forms will be written; one will be for resident participation in the ethnographic study; two will be for permission to be photographed (resident and staff forms). A copy of the resident participation informed consent form can be found in Appendix B.

All study participants will be asked to sign informed consents prior to formal interviews and photograph sessions. Confidentiality of the subjects and informants (staff) will be maintained by not identifying them by name. Data will be recorded with special code names, so that there is no link between these codes and the subject's identity. Names of the subjects and informants will be known only to the investigator, who will hold this information in the strictest confidence, coded, and securely stored in a locked file (in the home of the investigator) for a period of not less than 3 years.

Once agreeing to participate in this study, all participants will be informed that they are free to withdraw from the study at any time. They will also be informed that if the content of the interviews causes emotional discomfort or stress, they are free to terminate the interview at that time and also are at liberty to refuse to answer any question. All participants will be informed that their participation in this study or their wish not to participate will not, in any way, affect their status at Sunrise Manor.

Nursing Implications

Being homeless is accompanied by a multitude of problems. Having AIDS is saturated with its own distinctive set of physical, psychological, and social puzzles. The medical, especially the neurologic, problems that are common in AIDS further increase and aggravate the existing gravity of the person's life prior to becoming homeless.

Being a homeless PWA is a "contemporary condition," and it is anticipated that the description derived from this ethnography will present new dilemmas for health care professionals and society. Finding answers to such dilemmas will necessitate that the nurse look beyond the health care setting for practical answers.

As the numbers of AIDS cases multiply, the need for facilities such as Sunrise Manor will undoubtedly increase. AIDS is not a problem that lends itself to simple or immediate solutions, and descriptions of homeless PWAs in other parts of the country are necessary to understand the magnitude and intricacies of the AIDS dilemma. The intent of this study is to establish the first description of what it is like to be a homeless PWA living in a congregate facility from the PWAs' perspective. The findings from this investigation will enhance the knowledge base of the nursing profession with regard to the needs of this population and assist with planning appropriate interventions.

Appendix A: Interview Schedule

1. What is it like for you to live in Sunrise Manor?
2. What was it like for you before you moved in?
3. How are things here compared to where you were before?
4. How do you spend the day?

Appendix B: Informed Consent Form—Living in Sunrise Manor

1. *Purpose* You are being asked to participate in a research study in which you will be asked to describe your thoughts and feelings as a person

living in Sunrise Manor. The reason for conducting this study is to understand what it is like to live in Sunrise Manor and to determine how the experience can be made more beneficial to the residents.

2. *Procedure* The study will consist of three to five interviews that the investigator will conduct over a period of 2 to 3 months. The interviews will last approximately 60 minutes. You will be asked to respond to questions about what it is like to live in Sunrise Manor and what things were like for you before you moved in. The interviews will be tape recorded and the tape recordings will be erased once the tapes have been typed. At your request, the tape recorder will be turned off at any time during the interview(s). Toward the end of this study, a request may be made to take photographs of resident activities in Sunrise Manor. The photographs will be used to assist in describing the residence and its social activities. The photographs will not be published or displayed in any manner. The photographs will be destroyed at the end of the study. Only persons granting permission to be included in photographs will be.

3. *Risks* There are no anticipated physical risks involved by participating in this study. If you feel that the content of an interview is causing you feelings of stress or emotional discomfort, please know that you may end the interview.

4. *Benefits* There is no direct benefit to you for participating in this study. The results of this study may help health care providers gain understanding and make necessary changes to improve your living environment while in Sunrise Manor.

5. *Confidentiality* Names will not be used in the reporting of any information you tell the investigator. All information that refers to, or can be identified with you, will remain confidential to the extent permitted by law. The results of this study will be reported as group results.

6. *Participation is voluntary* Your participation in this study is voluntary. If you decide to participate and later decide that you do not wish to continue, you may at any time withdraw your consent and stop your participation, without affecting your status at Sunrise Manor. You may refuse to answer any question without affecting your status at Sunrise Manor or your continued participation in this study.

7. *Whom to contact for answers* If there are any questions at any time regarding this study or your participation in it, you are always free to consult with the Investigator [Suzan Jaffe: (305) 000–0000].

8. I have read and received a copy of this informed consent form.

SIGNATURE OF INVESTIGATOR, DATE   SIGNATURE OF PARTICIPANT, DATE

SIGNATURE OF WITNESS _____   DATE _____

Bibliography

Cassens, B. J. 1985. "Social Consequences of AIDS." *Annals of Internal Medicine,* 103: 768–771.

Center for Disease Control (CDC). October 1989. *HIV / AIDS Surveillance Report.*

Denker, A. L. 1986. "An Ethnography of AIDS Care." Unpublished manuscript, University of Miami, School of Nursing.

Dewar, H. 1989. "Homeless Don't Fit Image." *Miami Herald,* April 27, Section B: 1B–2B.

Freidson, E. 1974. *Profession of Medicine: A Study of the Sociology of Applied Knowledge.* New York: Dodd & Mead.

Goffman, E. 1963. *Stigma.* New York: Simon and Schuster.

Kelly, J. A., J. S. St Lawrence, et al. (1987). "Stigmatization of AIDS Patients by Physicians." *American Journal of Public Health,* 77(7): 789–791.

Leininger, M. M. 1985. *Qualitative Research Methods in Nursing.* New York: Grune & Stratton.

Lincoln, Y. S., & E. G. Guba. 1985. *Naturalistic Inquiry.* Beverly Hills, CA: Sage Publications.

McCombie, S. C. 1986. "The Cultural Impact of the 'AIDS' Test: The American Experience." *Social Science Medicine,* 23(5): 455–459.

Shoham, S. G., & G. Rahav. 1970. *The Mark of Cain.* St. Lucia: University of Queensland Press.

Spradley, J. P. 1979. *The Ethnographic Interview.* New York: Holt, Rinehart & Winston.

D ___ Guidelines for Evaluating a Research Report

A. The problem
   1. The problem is clearly identified.
   2. The problem is researchable (data can be collected and analyzed).
   3. It is feasible to conduct research on the problem.
   4. The problem is significant to nursing.
   5. Background information on the problem is presented.
B. Review of the literature
   1. The review is relevant to the study.
   2. The review is adequate in relation to the problem.
   3. References are current.
   4. Documentation of references is clear and complete.
   5. The relationship of the problem to previous research is clear.
   6. There is a range of opinions and varying points of view about the problem.
   7. The organization of the review is logical.
   8. The review concludes with a brief summary of the literature and its implications for the problem.
C. Theoretical or conceptual framework
   1. It is applicable to the research.
   2. It is clearly developed.
   3. It is useful for clarifying pertinent concepts and relationships.

D. Statement of the purpose of the study
  1. The statement form is appropriate for the study: declarative statement, question, hypothesis(es).
  2. The statement form is clear as to:
    a. what the researcher plans to do.
    b. where the data will be collected.
    c. from whom the data will be collected.
  3. Each hypothesis states an expected relationship or difference between two variables.
  4. There is a clear empirical or theoretical rationale for each hypothesis.
E. Definition of terms
  1. Relevant terms are clearly defined, either directly, operationally, or theoretically.
F. Data collection
  1. Study subjects
    a. The target population is clearly described.
    b. The sample size and major characteristics are appropriate (the sample is representative).
    c. The method for choosing the sample is appropriate.
    d. The sample size is adequate for the problem being investigated.
  2. Data collection instruments
    a. Instruments are appropriate for problem and method.
    b. Rationale for choosing instruments is discussed.
    c. Each instrument is described as to purpose, content, strengths, and weaknesses.
    d. Instrument validity is discussed.
    e. Instrument reliability is discussed.
    f. If the instrument was developed for the study:
      1. rationale for development is discussed.
      2. procedures in development are discussed.

3. reliability is discussed.
4. validity is discussed.
3. Procedures
   a. The research approach is appropriate.
   b. Steps in the data collection procedure are described clearly and concisely.
   c. The data collection procedure is appropriate for the study.
   d. Protection of human rights is assured.
   e. The study is replicable from the information provided.
   f. Appropriate limitations of the study are stated.
   g. Significant assumptions are stated.
G. Data analysis
   1. The choice of statistical procedures is appropriate.
   2. Statistical procedures are correctly applied to the data.
   3. Tables, charts, and graphs are clear and well labeled.
   4. Tables, charts, and graphs are pertinent.
   5. Tables, charts, and graphs reflect reported findings.
   6. Tables, charts, and graphs are clearly discussed in the text.
H. Conclusions and recommendations
   1. Results are discussed in relation to the study's purpose.
   2. Results are discussed in relation to the theoretical or conceptual framework.
   3. Interpretations are based on the data.
   4. Generalizations are warranted by the results.
   5. Conclusions are based on the data.
   6. Conclusions are clearly stated.
   7. Recommendations are plausible and relevant.
I. Summary
   1. The summary restates the problem.
   2. The summary restates the methodology.

Yes   No   N/A

    3. The summary restates the major findings
and conclusions.
    4. The summary is clear and concise.

J. Other considerations
    1. The investigator(s) is qualified.
    2. The title is appropriate, accurately reflecting the problem.
    3. The abstract presents a concise summary of the study.
    4. The article is well organized and flows logically.
    5. Grammar, sentence structure, and punctuation are correct.
    6. References and bibliography are accurate and complete.

Use the following criteria to rate the scientific merit of the report:

Rating	Criteria
4	Critique indicates that overall, the study satisfies the basic requirements of scientific research.
3	Critique indicates that overall, the study satisfies the basic requirements of scientific research with the following exceptions:
2	Critique indicates that overall, the study does not satisfy the basic requirements for scientific research with the following exceptions:
1	Critique indicates that overall, the study does not satisfy the basic requirements of scientific research.

Rating _____

E ___ Preparing a Research Proposal

The senior author of this book formulated the following step-by-step guidelines that are useful in writing proposals for both quantitative and qualitative studies. Components of the guidelines may be modified for qualitative proposals. For example, in grounded theory design there may be no review of the literature before collecting the data related to the study problem. There also will be no theoretical framework, since the purpose of the grounded theory approach is to develop theory. A proposal for ethnographic research may require a detailed presentation of the qualifications of the researcher or researchers involved in the study, since they are the primary data collection instruments. *The future tense should be used in writing the proposal.*

Writing the Problem Statement Section of a Research Proposal

The introductory phase of a research proposal entails a discussion of the following elements of research:

1. Background and rationale for selecting the study problem, including significance of the problem to nursing and the relevance of the problem to nursing.
2. Review of related literature.
3. Placement of the problem within a conceptual or theoretical framework, if appropriate.
4. Statement of the purpose of the study followed by definitions of all the terms used in the statement of the purpose.

In this initial section of the research proposal, the study's general subject area is discussed and then narrowed down to the focus of the study. It concludes with the research question, which should be stated in declarative form. Enough background material should be presented to acquaint the reader with the problem's importance. The rationale for selecting the problem should be discussed, as well as the study's significance and its contributions to nursing's scientific knowledge base. If appropriate, the problem should be placed in a theoretical or conceptual framework and a review of the relevant literature should be presented. The purpose of the study should be stated in a clearly defined statement as a declarative sentence, a question, or as a hypothesis (hypotheses) to be tested. All terms should be defined either directly, operationally, or theoretically. Recommendations for locating and using pertinent materials for the literature review are included at the end of this appendix.

Writing the Plan for the Data Collection Section of a Research Proposal

This part of a research proposal entails a discussion of the following:

1. The research approach to be used for the study.
2. Plans for the selection of the study subjects (sampling).
3. Techniques for data collection.
4. Procedures for data collection.
5. Assumptions of the study.
6. Limitations of the study.

In writing this section of the research proposal, the research approach is described as either historical, descriptive, or experimental. Plans for selection of the study subjects are specified in terms of the target population, kinds and numbers of study subjects, and the sampling approach and method (if applicable). Techniques for collecting the data are described in relation to the purpose of the study. The measuring instruments for a quantitative study are described and discussed in terms of their reliability, validity, and usability. An experimental study should also include a description of the experimental design. Steps in the procedure for data collection should be listed in chronologic order with attention to the protection of human rights. Any explicit assumptions that would significantly affect the study should be stated. Finally, the limitations of the study should be listed.

Writing the Data Analysis Section of a Research Proposal

It is important to formulate a plan for data analysis in the planning stage of the research study and to describe this plan in detail in the research proposal. This ensures that the researcher will collect the data in a form that facilitates analysis. The data analysis plan should be appropriate to the problem under investigation and to the methodology of the study. The method for tabulating and organizing the data for quantitative studies should be clearly presented, along with a description of appropriate statistical procedures to be applied and the rationale for selecting them.

Skeleton outlines or dummy statistical tables, charts, and graphs provide a format for analyzing the variables being investigated and may lead to additional ideas for data analysis. Although the best plans for analysis may turn out later to be incomplete or somewhat inappropriate, a carefully formulated plan for data analysis established prior to the actual data collection should result in higher quality research studies and can also eliminate much distress on the part of the researcher.

Qualitative researchers should also establish their data analysis plan before beginning their studies. Because of the nature of qualitative data, the plan for analysis may not be as complete as in a quantitative study. Still, planning ahead can facilitate data analysis later.

Further Notes

In addition to the criteria already discussed you may want to include a timetable for the various steps to follow when carrying out the research proposal, as well as an estimate of the expenses associated with the research. Research proposals written for funding require that a budget of projected expenses be included. Guidelines for funding such proposals are very specific regarding the budget information that must be included.

The title of a research proposal should accurately reflect the relationship between the variables being studied and the population of the study. The title can be most easily formulated from the information in the purpose of the study section and should reflect this purpose well enough to communicate it to others. Ask yourself if someone reading the title in an index would know what your study is about. A well-formulated proposal title can usually serve as the title for the final report of the study.

Now that you have a tentative draft of the major sections of your research proposal, reread the draft to ensure you have a logical development of ideas within each section and throughout the proposal. You may want to exchange your proposal with a colleague and use the following guidelines for evaluating a research proposal.

Guidelines for Evaluating a Research Proposal

Title of research proposal:

A. Statement of the problem
   1. Introduction presents study's general subject area and narrows the focus to a specific problem area.
   2. Enough background material is presented to acquaint the reader with the problem's importance.
   3. The problem is important enough that it will contribute to general knowledge in the nursing field.

4. The problem is novel and/or the study is timely.
5. It is feasible to conduct research on the problem.

B. Literature Review
1. An adequate survey of the literature has been made on the problem.
2. The literature references are pertinent to the problem.
3. The literature citations are well documented.
4. The organization of related evidence is logical.
5. The literature review is summarized.

C. Theoretical or conceptual framework
1. Applicable to the research being done.
2. Useful for clarifying concepts and relationships contained in the research.

D. Statement of the purpose of the study
1. Contains a clear statement of
   a. what the researcher intends to do (i.e., observe, describe, classify, and so on).
   b. where the data will be collected (study setting).
   c. from whom the data will be collected (study subjects).
2. Statement form is appropriate for the study problem (declarative statement, question, hypothesis).

E. Definition of terms
1. The terms in the study are defined so there is no question in the reader's mind as to what the researcher means.

F. Plan for data collection
1. The research approach (design)—historical, descriptive, experimental—is described and appropriate for the purpose of the study.
2. Study subjects
   a. The target population is described.
   b. The kinds and numbers of subjects are appropriate.
   c. The sampling approach (method) is appropriate.
3. Techniques for data collection
   a. The data collection instrument is appropriate for the research problem.
   b. The data can be quantified for analysis.
   c. Plans for determining the instrument's reliability are included.
   d. Plans for establishing the instrument's validity are included.
   e. The instrument's limitations are recognized.
   f. Plans for pretesting the instrument are included (as applicable).
4. Procedure for data collection
   a. Steps in the procedure are stated clearly and concisely.
   b. Data collection procedure is appropriate for the study.
   c. Protection of human rights is assured.

5. Assumptions underlying the study are stated if significant.
6. Study's limitations are appropriate.
G. Plan for data analysis
1. Data analysis is consistent with sample and instrument(s).
2. Statistical procedures are appropriate for the data.
3. Rationale for statistical procedure is correctly formulated.
4. Dummy charts, graphs, and tables are included.
H. Additional components
1. The title of the research proposal is appropriate.
2. Correct grammar is used.
3. Correct spelling and punctuation are used.
4. Reference format
   a. Citation (footnote) references are listed in consistent and correct format.
   b. Bibliographic entries are listed in consistent and correct format.

Recommendations for Locating Pertinent Materials for the Literature Review

It is extremely important for the researcher to familiarize him or herself with the available library resources before beginning the literature review. The time initially spent familiarizing oneself with these resources ultimately saves much valuable time. It is helpful to get a written guide that explains the resources and services of the library and the procedures to follow as well as participating in a guided tour of the library to learn how to use the library to its fullest extent.

Interlibrary loans are designed to help obtain references not available in your own library. Computerized literature searches such as MEDLARS or MEDLINE should be investigated. MEDLARS (Medical Literature Analysis and Retrieval System) is the computerized literature retrieval service of the National Library of Medicine in Bethesda, Maryland. MEDLARS contains millions of references to journal articles and books in the health sciences published after 1965. MEDLINE (MEDLARS on-line), the retrieval capability of MEDLARS, contains citations and selected abstracts from approximately 3000 journals published in the United States and foreign countries. It has hundreds of thousands of references to biomedical journal articles published in the current year and the 3 preceding years.

Table E-1 lists some, but not all, of the available computerized literature searches. These data bases are valuable sources for locating pertinent references.

Indexes and abstracts can help identify relevant references. Indexes are

Table E-1. Computerized Literature Searches

Data Base	Content
AVLINE, CATLINE	Audiovisuals and books in the biomedical sciences
BIOETHICS	Ethics
BIOSIS	Biological research
CANCERLIT	Cancer literature
CANCERPROJ	Cancer-related research projects
CHEMLINE	Dictionary of chemicals
CLINPROT	Clinical cancer protocols
DIOGENES	FDA and drug information
DIRLINE	Directory of information resources
EMBASE	Formerly *Excerpta Medica*
ERIC	Educational Resources Information Center, U.S. Office of Education
HEALTH	Health care aspects, such as planning
HEALTH INSTRUMENT FILE	Describes behavioral instruments used by nurse researchers
HISTLINE	History of medicine and related sciences
PSYCINFO	Psychology and related literature, including nursing
SOCABS	*Sociological Abstracts,* American Sociological Association
TOXLINE	Toxicologic information

lists of books and articles, or the contents of a book, whereas abstracts present the main ideas of articles and books.

The following indexes are useful:

1. The *Cumulative Index to Nursing and Allied Health Literature,* published continuously since 1956, indexes approximately 250 English-language journals in nursing and allied health sciences. The index also contains selected articles from popular magazines and some biomedical journals from *Index Medicus.*

2. *Hospital Literature Index,* published quarterly by the American Hospital Association, selectively indexes approximately 600 English-language journals on health care administration and planning.

3. *Index Medicus,* a government publication under the auspices of the National Library of Medicine, surveys over 2600 international biomedical journals, of which several are nursing journals.

4. *International Nursing Index,* published quarterly by the American Journal of Nursing Company in cooperation with the National Library of Medicine, surveys approximately 200 domestic and foreign journals, in addition to nursing articles from over 2600 non-nursing journals.

The following abstracts are helpful:

1. *Dissertation Abstracts International* contains abstracts of doctoral dissertations in the humanities and social sciences, the sciences, engineering, and nursing.
2. *Psychological Abstracts,* published by the American Psychological Association, abstracts the international literature on psychology and related disciplines and contains categories related to nursing and nursing education.
3. *Sociological Abstracts* contains abstracts of the international literature in sociology and has sections on nursing.

The following indexes and abstracts are the other major sources commonly used by nurse researchers:

Abstracts of Health Care Management Studies
American Journal of Nursing: Annual and Cumulative Indexes
Biological Abstracts
Bioresearch Abstracts
Child Development Abstracts
Education Index
ERIC (Educational Resources Information Center)
Excerpta Medica
International Index
Nursing Outlook: Annual and Cumulative Indexes
Nursing Research: Annual and Cumulative Indexes
Nutrition Abstracts
Public Health, Social Medicine and Hygiene
Readers' Guide to Periodical Literature
Research Grants Index
Science Citation Index

In addition to indexes and abstracts, compilations of measuring instruments can be helpful in identifying relevant references and locating appropriate measuring instruments. The following compilations are specifically related to nursing research:

Clayton, G. M., and M. Broom. 1989. *Instruments for Use in Nursing Education Research.* No. 15-2248. New York: National League for Nursing.
Frank-Stromberg, M. (1992). *Instruments for Clinical Nursing Research.* Boston: Jones and Bartlett.
Ward, M. J., and C. Lindeman. Eds. 1978. *Instruments for Measuring*

Nursing Practice and Other Care Variables. 2 vols. DHEW Publication No. HRA 78-53. Washington, DC: U.S. Government Printing Office.

Ward, M. J., and M. Fetter. 1979. *Instruments for Use in Nursing Education Research.* Boulder, CO: Western Interstate Commission for Higher Education.

A list of selected sources for locating measuring instruments that are not specifically related to nursing research follow:

Buros, O. K., Ed. 1970, 1975. *Personality Tests and Review.* 2 vols. Highland Park, NJ: Gryphon Press.

Chun, K. T., S. Cobb, and J. French, Jr. 1975. *Measures for Psychological Assessment.* Ann Arbor: University of Michigan Institute for Social Research.

Goldman, B., and J. Saunders. 1974. *Directory of Unpublished Experimental Measures.* 2 vols. New York: Behavioral Publications.

Johnson, O. 1976. *Tests and Measurements in Child Development: Handbook 11.* 2 vols. San Francisco: Jossey-Bass.

Keyser, D. J., and R. C. Sweetland, Eds. 1987. *Test Critiques.* Kansas City: Test Corporation of America.

Miller, D., Ed. 1991. *Handbook of Research Design and Social Measurement,* 5th ed. Newbury Park, CA: Sage.

Mitchell, J. V., Jr., Ed. 1985. *Mental Measurements Yearbook,* 9th ed. Lincoln: University of Nebraska Press.

Murphy, L., J. C. Conoley, and J. C. Impara. Eds. 1994. *Tests in Print IV.* Lincoln: University of Nebraska Press.

Newmark, C. S. 1989. *Major Psychological Assessment Instruments.* Boston: Allyn and Bacon.

Reeder, L., L. Ramacher, and S. Gorelnik. 1976. *Handbook of Scales and Indices of Health Behavior.* Santa Monica, CA: Goodyear Publishing Company.

Shaw, M. E., and J. M. Wright. 1967. *Scales for the Measurement of Attitudes.* New York: McGraw-Hill.

Strauss, M., and B. W. Brown. 1978. *Family Measurement Techniques: Abstracts of Published Instruments, 1935 to 1974,* revised. Minneapolis: University of Minnesota Press.

Sweetland, R. C., and D. J. Keyser, Eds. 1991. *Tests: A Comprehensive Reference for Assessments in Psychology, Education and Business,* 3rd ed. Austin, TX: Pro-Ed.

Health and Psychosocial Instruments (HaPI) CD ROM

The Internet is an important source for locating information. This is an international computer network that can help researchers locate information quickly from almost anywhere in the world. Most institutions of higher learning are connected to the Internet; the computer services department should be able to help you get on-line to search for topics that interest you.

It is preferable to obtain reference material from primary (original) sources rather than secondary (not original) sources. This minimizes error and allows the researcher to analyze the material. Articles you plan to quote directly should be photocopied to reduce citation errors. You should also plan to photocopy all tables and charts that you cite so that you have the complete information when writing the report.

After locating references that are pertinent to your topic, you should begin with the latest one since it may contain additional references from previous research. Read the abstract of the article and the summary, or both, to see if the article is pertinent to your topic. Then scan the article, noting the important points. Plan to use separate index cards (4 × 6 is a convenient size) to record useful information. A separate index card for each reference helps organize the materials when you are ready to write up the literature review.

The index card should contain the following information:

1. A complete record of bibliographic references in the format of the style manual required by your department. This record saves you time when you write the bibliography for your proposal.

2. The complete call number for a source in case you need to recheck it.

3. A coding system for each reference. When using this coding system, mark such factors as relevance to your study, type of article, and whatever else that is helpful for your research. For example, information on the relevance of references could be coded as R + (very relevant), R (relevant), or R − (less relevant). Information concerning the type of reference could be coded as RS (research study) or V (an article expressing the author's viewpoint).

4. A summary of the reference that lists its essential points and notes the important or unusual aspects of the article. If you quote directly from the article, copy the quotation word for word, being careful to note if it is a direct quotation.

5. A note that indicates if a reference is a primary or secondary source. Primary sources are first-hand information, not interpretations. Secondary sources are interpretations of, or references to, primary sources.

After thoroughly investigating the relevant references, you need to organize them in order to write the literature review. To refresh your memory, review the notes on each card and discard irrelevant references. Include only those references that you used to substantiate your research. Next, make a tentative outline showing the relationships among the topics. Then analyze your cards, putting them into the appropriate categories of the outline. For each category, analyze the similarities and differences between the references. Summarize those references that state essentially the same thing—for example, "Smith (1987), Brown (1988), and Green (1990) report that . . ." Include studies that show results contradictory to those you expect to find from your study. When organizing the literature review, discuss the references that are least related to the problem first, progressing to the most relevant references. Conclude the review with a brief summary of the main points, general conclusions, and implications.

Glossary

Abstract A concise summary of a study.

Accidental sampling Nonprobability sampling method in which the sampling units are selected because they are available to the investigator at the time of data collection. Also called *convenience sampling.*

Alternate forms reliability Method of determining reliability in which two different forms of an instrument are administered to the same individuals and the two sets of scores are then correlated. Also called *equivalent forms reliability.*

Analysis of covariance (ANCOVA) Parametric statistical test to determine the differences between the means of two or more groups by removing the effects of one or more confounding variables.

Analysis of variance (ANOVA) Parametric statistical test to determine the differences between the means of two or more groups.

Anonymity Protection of the rights of the study subjects so that the respondents are not directly linked to their responses.

Applied research Research conducted to generate new knowledge that can be applied in practical settings without undue delay.

Assumption A statement whose correctness or validity is taken for granted.

Attrition Loss of subjects during a research study.

Basic research Research designed to formulate theory rather than be utilized for immediate application.

Case studies In-depth studies of individuals or small groups.

Chi-square (χ^2) A statistical technique used to determine if observed frequencies differ from expected frequencies.

Cliometrics Use of statistical analysis in historical research.

Cluster sampling A probability sample in which the cluster is the primary sampling unit. Clusters consist of groups that have the same characteristic(s).

Concept A single idea (often one word) that represents several related ideas (e.g., *grief*).

Conceptual framework Discussion of the relationship of concepts that underlie the study problem and support the rationale (reason) for conducting the study.

Confidentiality   Responses of study subjects are not linked with the individuals who provided them when the study results are communicated.

Confounding variables   Variables that may interfere with the direct causal relationship of independent variables to dependent variables.

Construct   Hypothetical grouping of abstract concepts (prejudice, intelligence).

Construct validity   The degree to which a measuring instrument measures a specific hypothetical trait, such as intelligence.

Content analysis   ". . . the technique that provides a systematic means of measuring the frequency, order, or intensity of words, phrases or sentences" [1].

Content validity   A method for determining the validity of a measuring instrument that utilizes the consensus of a judge panel of experts. The panel agrees that the measuring instrument measures what it is said to measure.

Control   Elimination or reduction of extraneous variables that could influence the dependent variable under investigation.

Control group   The group in which the experimental treatment is not introduced.

Convenience sampling   See *Accidental sampling*.

Correlation   The strength of the quantifiable relationship between two or more variables.

Correlation coefficient   The number that represents the strength of the quantifiable relationship between two or more variables.

Criterion-related validity   The general term that includes concurrent and predictive validity. Refers to the relationship of the measuring instrument to some already known external criterion or other valid instrument.

Criterion variable   A preestablished measure of success. Sometimes called the *dependent variable*.

Cross-sectional study   A research technique in which data are collected at a certain point in time.

Datum   A unit of information (plural: *data*).

Debriefing   Providing subjects of the study with information about the study after the study has been concluded.

Deductive   Method of reasoning that moves from the general to the specific.

Delphi technique   A research methodology for predicting or emphasizing the main concerns of a group.

Dependent variable   The variable that changes as the independent variable is manipulated by the researcher; sometimes called the *criterion variable*.

Descriptive research approach Research approach that is present-oriented and designed to answer questions based on the ongoing events of the present.

Descriptive statistics Statistics used to describe and summarize data.

Direct definition Definition of a term taken from the dictionary.

Double blind study Experimental strategy in which neither the subjects nor those who collect the data know which subjects are in the experimental group and which subjects are in the control group.

Empirical evidence Data gathered to generate new knowledge. It must be rooted in objective reality and gathered directly or indirectly through human senses.

Empirical generalization A principle derived from empirical evidence.

Ethnography Inductive research approach for in-depth investigation of a culture or cultures in which data related to the members of the culture are collected, analyzed, and described.

Experimental research approach Research approach in which the independent variable(s) is manipulated under controlled conditions to determine the effect on the dependent variable(s); also characterized by random assignment of study subjects to treatment conditions.

Exploratory study (pilot study) A preliminary study used to determine strengths and weaknesses of a planned project; may also be used as the basis of future studies.

Ex post facto research Type of research design in which the independent variable is not manipulated because changes in the independent variable have already occurred prior to the study.

External criticism The evaluation of the validity of historical data.

Extraneous variable Uncontrolled variables outside the purpose of the study that influence the study's results.

Face validity A subjective method for determining validity of a measuring instrument. It is determined by inspection of the items to see that the instrument contains important items that measure the variables being studied.

Frequency distribution The arrangement of the scores or values of characteristics from the highest to the lowest or in a systematic way.

Friedman two-way analysis of variance by ranks Nonparametric statistical test using ordinal-level data to determine whether related samples have come from the same population by determining mean ranks.

Generalizability   See *Inference.*

Grounded theory   Inductive research approach that generates the theoretical underpinnings of the research by "grounding" or basing the theory in the data being collected.

H₀   See *Null hypothesis.*

Hawthorne effect   Term used to describe the psychological reactions to the presence of the investigator, or to special treatment during a research study, which tend to alter the responses of the subject.

Historical research approach   Research approach that deals with what has happened in the past and how those happenings affect the present.

Hypothesis   A statement of predicted relationships between the variables under study; an educated or calculated guess by the researcher. It is the testable component of the research (plural: *hypotheses*).

Independent variable   The variable that is purposely manipulated or changed by the researcher; also called the *manipulated variable.*

Inductive   Method of reasoning that moves from the specific to the general.

Inference   Information gathered from a sample is generalized to a population.

Inferential statistics   Statistical tests used to make inferences (generalizations) to the larger population from which the sample was drawn.

Informed consent   Voluntary agreement by a study subject to participate in a research study after being informed about the study and the rights of the subjects who participate.

Institutional Review Board (IRB)   A committee appointed by an agency to review research being conducted within the agency to ensure protection of the rights of subjects participating in a research study.

Internal criticism   The evaluation of the reliability or accuracy of what is stated in a historical document.

Interrater reliability   Method for determining reliability in which the strength of agreement between the observations made by two or more observers is determined. Also called *interobserver reliability.*

Interval data scale   Data based on a scale that has equal intervals.

Interview   Verbal questioning of respondents by the investigator in order to collect data. Requires interaction between people.

Judgment sampling   See *Purposive sampling.*

Kruskal-Wallis one-way analysis of variance by ranks   A nonparametric statistical test that ranks ordinal-level data to determine whether independent samples were drawn from the same continuous population.

Level of significance   The probability level used to reject the null hypothesis.

Likert scale   A scale for rating attitudes in which each statement usually has five possible responses: strongly agree, agree, uncertain, disagree, strongly disagree.

Longitudinal study   A research design in which data are collected from the same subjects over a period of time.

Manipulated variable   See *Independent variable.*

Mann-Whitney U   Nonparametric statistical test that uses ordinal data (ranks) to determine if two independent samples have been drawn from the same population.

Mean   The arithmetic average.

Measures of central tendency   See *Mean, Median, Mode, Standard deviation.*

Median   The number above which 50 percent of the observations fall.

MEDLARS (Medical Literature Analysis and Retrieval System)   The computerized literature retrieval service of the National Library of Medicine.

MEDLINE   A computerized data base that references biomedical journal articles.

Meta-analysis   "The statistical analysis of a large collection of results from individual studies for the purpose of integrating the findings into a single, generalizable finding" [2].

Mode   The most frequently occurring score or number value.

Multiple analysis of variance (MANOVA)   Parametric statistical test to determine interaction effects between two or more independent variables and two or more dependent variables.

Nominal data scale   Data that can be separated only into mutually exclusive categories.

Nonparametric statistics   "A general class of inferential statistics that does not involve rigorous assumptions about the distribution of the critical variables: most often used when the data are measured on the nominal or ordinal scales" [3].

Nonprobability sampling   Sampling approach in which the investigator has no ability to estimate the probability that each element of the

population will be included in the sample, or even that it has some
chance of being included.

Normal curve   A theoretical bell-shaped curve with most measurement
clustered about the center and a few measurements at the extreme
ends.

Null hypothesis (H₀)   The most commonly used method of stating the
way the relationship between the variables being studied will be
tested. The null hypothesis is stated as follows: "There is no statistically significant difference between the experimental and the control
group." Also termed *statistical hypothesis.*

Nursing research   Research conducted to answer questions or find solutions to problems specifically related to nursing. It has the purpose of
developing an organized body of scientific knowledge unique to
nursing.

Observation   Watching and noting actions and reactions.

Operational definition   The researcher's definition of a term that provides a description of the method for studying the concept by citing
the necessary operations (manipulations and observations) to be used.

Opinionnaire   A questionnaire designed to elicit opinions.

Ordinal data scale   Data that are ordered, but for which there is no
zero starting point, and the intervals between individual data are not
equal. *Big, bigger,* and *biggest* are ordinal data.

Parametric statistics   ". . . a class of inferential statistics that involves
(a) assumptions about the distribution of the variables, (b) the estimation of a parameter, and (c) the use of interval measures" [4].

Participant observation   Observation techniques in which the observer becomes a participant in the situation being observed.

Pearson r (Pearson product-moment correlation coefficient)   A
frequently used correlation statistic. Correlation coefficients expressed as r's range from −1 to +1.

Percentile rank   Descriptive statistic indicating the point below which
a percentage of scores occurs.

Phenomenology   Inductive research approach based on the philosophy
of phenomenology, which proposes to understand the whole human
being through "the lived experience."

Pilot study   See *Exploratory study.*

Population   See *Target population.*

Population element   A single unit or member of the target population.

Pretest   (1) The process of testing out the effectiveness of a measuring
instrument in gathering appropriate data. (2) In an experimental

study, the data collection procedure prior to the experimental phase of the study.

Primary source First-hand information obtained from original material; not interpretive or hearsay information.

Probability sampling Sampling approach in which the investigator is able to specify, for each population element, the probability that it will be included in the sample. That is, there is a *known* probability of each element being included in the sample.

Projective tests Psychological tests that require the subjects to respond to ambiguous situations.

Protocol See *Research-based clinical protocol.*

Purposive sampling Nonprobability sampling method in which subjects are selected according to specific criteria established by the investigator. Also called *judgmental sampling.*

Qualitative data Data characterized by words (*pale, cyanotic,* and so on).

Quantitative data Data characterized by numbers.

Quasi-experimental research Research approach in which the independent variable is manipulated to determine the effect on the dependent variable, but subjects are not randomly assigned to treatment conditions.

Questionnaire A paper-and-pencil data collection instrument that is completed by the study subjects themselves to elicit their attitudes or feelings.

Quota sampling Nonprobability sampling method in which the investigator specifies a percentage for subjects' characteristics to be included in the sample to ensure adequate representation of those characteristics.

r See *Pearson r.*

Randomization Assignment of subjects to treatment conditions in such a manner that each population element is assigned by chance alone rather than by some purposive method.

Random sampling See *Simple random sampling* or *Stratified random sampling.*

Range The distribution of scores from the lowest to highest; the high score minus the low score.

Rating scale A scale that allows respondents to make a qualitative judgment. Rating scales yield ordinal data.

Ratio data scale Data based on a scale that has equal intervals and an absolute zero starting point.

Reliability   The degree to which a measuring instrument obtains consistent results when it is reused.

Replication   Repeating a study using the same study design but different study subjects.

Research   A scientific process of inquiry and/or experimentation that involves purposeful, systematic, and rigorous collection, analysis, and interpretation of data in order to gain new knowledge or add to the existing body of scientific knowledge.

Research-based clinical protocol   A written document that organizes and transforms research-based knowledge so that it can be used to direct clinical practice activities.

Research hypothesis   Method of stating the hypothesis so that the relationship between the variables that the researcher expects as the study's outcome is specified.

Research utilization   Transferring research-based knowledge into actual practice.

Sample   A smaller part of the target population selected in such a way that the individuals in the sample represent (as nearly as possible) the characteristics of the target population.

Sampling   Process of selecting a sample from the target population.

Sampling unit   See *Population element.*

Scientific method   An orderly process that utilizes the principles of science and requires the use of certain sequential steps to acquire dependable information in the solving of problems.

Secondary source   An interpretive or hearsay source of data.

Serendipitous findings   Unplanned and unexpected discovery of significant results in a research study not related to the purpose of the study.

Simple random sampling   A probability sample in which the required number of sampling units is selected at random from the population in such a manner that each population element has an equal chance (probability) of being selected.

Single blind study   Experimental strategy carried out in either of two ways: (1) The study subjects know whether they are in the experimental or control group, but the data collectors do not know; (2) the data collectors know whether subjects are in the experimental or control group, but the subjects do not know.

Spearman's rho (r_s)   A nonparametric measure of correlation.

Split-half reliability   Method for determining reliability in which responses to a measuring instrument are divided in half, scored separately, and then correlated. Also called odd–even reliability.

Spurious correlations   Correlations that yield high relationship values, but where no relationship actually exists.

Standard deviation   The general indicator of dispersion from the mean.

Statistical hypothesis   See *Null hypothesis.*

Statistical inference   Statistical analysis that permits conclusions to be drawn about a population based on examination of only a portion (sample) of the population.

Statistics   The techniques used to assemble, describe, and make inferences from numerical data.

Stratified random sampling   A variation of the simple random sample in which the target population is divided into two or more strata (categories of the characteristic), and a simple random sample is taken from each stratum (category).

Structured interview   An interview that has a set series of questions.

Student's t-test   See *t-Test.*

Survey research   Collection of data about present conditions directly from the study subjects, usually by questionnaire or interview.

Symbols   Those signs used to substitute for whole words or concepts, such as χ^2 for chi-square or r for Pearson product-moment correlation coefficient.

Target population   The total group of individual people or things meeting the designated set of criteria of interest to the researcher.

***t*-Test**   A parametric statistical measure to determine the differences between the means of two groups.

Test of significance   Statistical test utilized to determine differences between groups.

Test–retest reliability   Method for determining reliability in which the same instrument is administered to the same individuals at different times and the two sets of scores are then correlated.

Test statistic (*T*)   A test similar to the chi-square test but which allows expected cell values to be as low as 1 in more than 20 percent of the cells.

Theoretical definition   Definition of a term using the specific language of the theory being used.

Theoretical framework   Discussion of one theory or interrelated theories being tested in order to support the rationale (reason) for conducting the study.

Theory   A set of statements, called *propositions,* that are stated in such a way as to form a logically interrelated deductive system. Used to summarize existing knowledge and to explain and/or predict phenomena and their relationships.

Type I error   Rejection of the null hypothesis when it should be accepted. Also called the *alpha error.*

Type II error   Acceptance of the null hypothesis when it should be rejected. Also called the *beta error.*

Unstructured interview   An interview that has a general framework for eliciting data but does not have a fixed pattern of questions.

Utilization   See *Research utilization.*

Validity   The extent to which a data-gathering instrument measures what it is supposed to measure by obtaining data relevant to what is being measured.

Variable   A multivalued entity. The attribute or characteristic under study that varies in some dimension.

Variance   The square of the standard deviation. It reflects the distance of individual scores from the mean.

χ^2 See *Chi-square.*

Z-score   A number reflecting the distance that an individual score is from the mean in standard deviation units. Also termed standard score.

References

1. Burns, N., and S. K. Grove. 1987. *The Practice of Nursing Research: Conduct, Critique and Utilization.* Philadelphia: W. B. Saunders, p. 743.
2. Lynn, M. R. 1989. "Meta-Analysis: Appropriate Tool for Integration of Nursing Research?" *Nursing Research,* 38 (September–October): 302.
3. Polit, D., and B. Hungler. 1995. *Nursing Research: Principles and Methods* 5th ed. Philadelphia: J. B. Lippincott, p. 647.
4. Ibid., pp. 648–649.

Index

Notes

Notes

Notes

Notes

Notes

Notes

Notes

Notes

Notes

Notes

Workbook

1 Becoming Acquainted with Nursing Research

1. List as many words as you can think of that describe the term research.

2. Locate a published article that is a report of a research study that interests you. Since not every article is a research article in the strictest sense, look for an article that has the following parts:

    (1) *Title* (often long—usually touches on the research content)
    (2) *Author(s) Name and Affiliation*
    (3) *Abstract* (a short summary at the beginning of the article)
    (4) *Introduction and Literature Review*
    (5) *Method* (or methodology)—discusses how the research was carried out
    (6) *Results* (or findings)—reports what happened
    (7) *Discussion* (what the results mean)
    (8) *References*

    If you are not sure that you have found a research article, check with your instructor.

3. Use the article to *discuss* how it fulfills the definition of research presented in Chapter 1.

    a. The study is a scientific process of inquiry and/or experimentation

b. The study involves systematic and rigorous collection of data

c. The study involves analysis and interpretation of data

d. The study was designed to gain new knowledge that has the potential to contribute to an organized body of scientific knowledge

e. What aspects of the study could contribute to improved nursing practice for better patient care?

f. Classify the study by research purpose. Is it basic or applied research? _____ Why?

g. Classify the study by research approach. Is it descriptive, experimental, or historical research? _____ Why?

4. Define nursing research as you now understand it.

5. List at least three patient care problems that you believe could be researched from a nursing focus.

6. It has been stated that nurses should conduct their own research into the practice and profession of nursing. Do you agree or disagree with this statement? Defend your answer.

2 Stages of the Research Process

1. Explain in your own words why the research process is a process for *scientific* inquiry.

2. Read the proposal in Appendix B so that you can see what information a research proposal contains and what a completed proposal looks like.

   a. Why does this proposal represent the *planning stage* of the research process rather than the *implementation stage?*

   b. Explain why this proposal is an example of the *descriptive research approach* as discussed in Chapter 1.

3. Explain why the research proposal in Appendix A is an example of the *historical research approach* as discussed in Chapter 1.

4. Reread the published research article you have chosen for the exercises in Chapter 1. Use Table 2-1 in Chapter 2 to systematically analyze the investigator(s) use of the research process rather than the problem-solving process.

3   The Quantitative and Qualitative Traditions of Inquiry

1. List three differences between quantitative and qualitative research.

2. Explain the following terms in your own words:

   a. numerical analysis

   b. control

   c. replication

   d. phenomenology

   e. grounded theory

   f. ethnography

3. Read the proposal in Appendix C. List three reasons why this proposal is an example of using a qualitative research strategy for scientific inquiry.

4. In the published research study you selected for the Workbook Activities for Chapters 1 and 2, did the investigator use a quantitative or a qualitative strategy? Fill in the following to answer the question:

The investigator used a _____ research strategy because the study has the following characteristics:

4 ___ Ethical Considerations for Protection of Human Subjects

1. List three reasons why ethical codes for the conduct of research are necessary.

2. Why should the following organizations have institutional review boards?

   a. A hospital

   b. A health department

   c. A hospice

3. How would these institutional review boards be similar and how might they differ?

4. Read the informed consent at the end of the qualitative research proposal (Appendix C). Discuss how the researcher included the six elements of informed consent discussed in Chapter 4.

5. For the published research study you read for the Workbook Activities in Chapters 1, 2, and 3, discuss the extent to which the author reported procedures for the protection of the subjects in the study.

5 Problem Selection and Statement

1. Identify a clinical nursing problem that could be improved if research findings were used. For example, teaching breast-feeding to primiparas, pain assessment in postoperative infants, patient-controlled analgesia after hysterectomy, or the effect of preoperative teaching on postoperative compliance to treatment.

   My clinical nursing problem is:

2. Complete the following library search exercise,* designed to assist you in locating the literature relevant to the clinical problem you identified in the previous activity. If your library has CD ROM search capabilities, use both textual references and the CD ROM database for your search. If you use computerized databases you may be able to combine terms.

   First, list as many key words as you can that might relate to your clinical nursing problem. For example, for the topic "teaching breast-feeding to primiparas," the following key words could be related:

   Primiparas
   Teaching
   Instruction
   Infants: feeding
   Infant nutrition
   Neonatal nursing
   Lactation
   Milk
   Bottle feeding
   Mothering
   Breast-feeding

*Adapted from P. Dempsey, "Improving Library Skills." *Nursing Research* (September–October) 5:390. Copyright 1977, American Journal of Nursing Company. Reproduced with permission.

Key words relating to my clinical nursing problem are:

1.   4.   7.   10.

2.   5.   8.   11.

3.   6.   9.   12.

Additional key words:

- Begin your library search by listing three complete references from the *Cumulative Index to Nursing and Allied Health Literature* (CINAHL) concerning your clinical nursing problem.

- Go to the *Index Medicus* and list two complete references related to your clinical nursing problem.

- Using *Excerpta Medica,* list two complete references related to your clinical nursing problem.

- List one complete reference from *Dissertation Abstracts* related to your clinical nursing problem.

- Use *Psychological Abstracts* to locate psychological studies related to your clinical nursing problem. List at least two complete references from this source.

- List at least *one book* that relates to your clinical nursing problem (include author, title, publication date, and library call number).

- Look in *Child Development Abstracts* to determine pediatric applications to your clinical nursing problem. List *one reference* if possible.

- If there are any geriatric implications for your clinical nursing problem, list one reference.

- List at least three references from nursing research journals related to your clinical nursing problem.

- If there are references in the following indexes related to your clinical nursing problem, list one from each source:

  a. *Hospital Literature Index*

  b. *International Nursing Index*

  c. *Readers' Guide to Periodical Literature*

- List at least three references from government documents related to your clinical nursing problem.

- There are many other abstracts and indexes available that might provide additional reference citations related to your clinical nursing problem. List at least three abstracts, indexes, or both, related to your clinical nursing problem in addition to those you have already used and cite one reference from each source.

- Investigate a computerized literature search (such as MEDLARS or MEDLINE) available to you through your library or through other sources to see how it can help you locate further references related to your clinical nursing problem. Discuss what you found out about these sources.

- If possible, enter the Internet and list at least two references from other libraries that relate to your clinical nursing problem. Identify the sources of these references.

- Investigate audiovisual holdings concerning the broad area of nursing and list the names of three films and videotapes or both.

3. The following activities will help you understand more about hypotheses. Read the following three hypotheses.

(1) Patients with slightly elevated blood pressure will have lower blood pressure after training in stress reduction techniques.
(2) Nurses caring for patients with AIDS have a higher level of anxiety than nurses caring for oncology patients.
(3) Primiparas whose husbands have received instruction in neonatal care have fewer adjustment problems with their infant(s) than those whose husbands have not received such instruction.

a. State the independent variable and dependent variable for each of these hypotheses.
Hypothesis (1):

Independent variable:

Dependent variable:

Hypothesis (2):

Independent variable:

Dependent variable:

Hypothesis (3):

Independent variable:

Dependent variable:

b. Now state each hypothesis in the null form.
Hypothesis (1):

Hypothesis (2):

Hypothesis (3):

    c. Write an operational definition for a term used in one of the null hypotheses you have just stated.

4. In these next activities, you will begin to learn the process for critically evaluating published research as described in Chapter 5. First, you will need to locate three of the research studies you identified in your literature search that are related to your clinical nursing problem. These studies should interest you enough to use them to learn the process of critical evaluation for the remainder of the course.

    Use the following questions to evaluate the problem selection and statement section for each of the studies you selected. If the author(s) did not include the information requested either say *no* or *not applicable.*

Study 1

Title

Author(s)

Publication information

    Journal

    Publication date

    Pages: From: _____ To: _____

A. The problem

    1. Has the author clearly identified the research problem? What is it?

2. Is the problem researchable, that is, can data be collected and analyzed?

3. Is it feasible to conduct research on the problem?

4. Is the problem significant to nursing?

5. Is background information on the problem presented?

B. Review of the literature

1. Is the review relevant to the study?

2. Is the review adequate in relation to the problem?

3. Are sources current?

4. Is documentation of sources clear and complete?

5. Is the relationship of the problem to previous research clear?

6. Is there a range of opinions and varying points of view about the problem?

7. Is the organization of the review logical?

8. Does the review conclude with a brief summary of the literature and its implications for the problem?

C. If there is a theoretical or conceptual framework

1. Is it applicable to the research?

2. Is it clearly developed?

3. Is it useful for clarifying pertinent concepts and relationships?

D. Statement of the purpose of the study

1. Is the statement form appropriate for the study: declarative statement, question, hypothesis(es)?

2. Is the statement form clear as to:

a. what the researcher planned to do?

b. where the data will be collected?

c. from whom the data will be collected?

3. Does each hypothesis state an expected relationship or difference between two variables?

4. Is there a clear empirical or theoretical rationale for each hypothesis?

E. Definition of terms

1. Is each relevant term clearly defined, either *directly, operationally, or theoretically?*

List the definition of each term and identify the type of definition used.

Study 2

Title

Author(s)

Publication information

Journal

Publication date

Pages: From: _____ To: _____

A. The problem

    1. Has the author clearly identified the research problem? What is it?

    2. Is the problem researchable, that is, can data be collected and analyzed?

    3. Is it feasible to conduct research on the problem?

    4. Is the problem significant to nursing?

    5. Is background information on the problem presented?

B. Review of the literature

    1. Is the review relevant to the study?

    2. Is the review adequate in relation to the problem?

    3. Are sources current?

4. Is documentation of sources clear and complete?

5. Is the relationship of the problem to previous research clear?

6. Is there a range of opinions and varying points of view about the problem?

7. Is the organization of the review logical?

8. Does the review conclude with a brief summary of the literature and its implications for the problem?

C. If there is a theoretical or conceptual framework

1. Is it applicable to the research?

2. Is it clearly developed?

3. Is it useful for clarifying pertinent concepts and relationships?

D. Statement of the purpose of the study

   1. Is the statement form appropriate for the study: declarative statement, question, hypothesis(es)?

   2. Is the statement form clear as to:

      a. what the researcher planned to do?

      b. where the data will be collected?

      c. from whom the data will be collected?

   3. Does each hypothesis state an expected relationship or difference between two variables?

   4. Is there a clear empirical or theoretical rationale for each hypothesis?

E. Definition of terms

   1. Is each relevant term clearly defined, either *directly, operationally,* or *theoretically?*

List the definition of each term and identify the type of definition used.

Study 3

Title

Author(s)

Publication information

Journal

Publication date

Pages: From: _____ To: _____

A. The problem

1. Has the author clearly identified the research problem? What is it?

2. Is the problem researchable, that is, can data be collected and analyzed?

3. Is it feasible to conduct research on the problem?

4. Is the problem significant to nursing?

5. Is background information on the problem presented?

B. Review of the literature

  1. Is the review relevant to the study?

  2. Is the review adequate in relation to the problem?

  3. Are sources current?

  4. Is documentation of sources clear and complete?

  5. Is the relationship of the problem to previous research clear?

  6. Is there a range of opinions and varying points of view about the problem?

  7. Is the organization of the review logical?

  8. Does the review conclude with a brief summary of the literature and its implications for the problem?

C. If there is a theoretical or conceptual framework

  1. Is it applicable to the research?

2. Is it clearly developed?

3. Is it useful for clarifying pertinent concepts and relationships?

D. Statement of the purpose of the study

1. Is the statement form appropriate for the study: declarative statement, question, hypothesis(es)?

2. Is the statement form clear as to:

   a. what the researcher planned to do?

   b. where the data will be collected?

   c. from whom the data will be collected?

3. Does each hypothesis state an expected relationship or difference between two variables?

4. Is there a clear empirical or theoretical rationale for each hypothesis?

E. Definition of terms

   1. Is each relevant term clearly defined, either *directly, operationally,* or *theoretically?*

     List the definition of each term and identify the type of definition used.

6 Data Collection

The following exercises are designed to help you better understand the data collection component of the research process and how it is applied to critical evaluation of research.

1. *Use the following procedure to select study subjects by simple random sampling:*

   The desired sample size for a quantitative study is 20 subjects selected from a target population of 40 elements. Select the subjects to be included in the sample by following this procedure:

   a. List the elements (names) of the target population.
   b. Number the names consecutively from 01 to 40.
   c. Arbitrarily select a two-digit column from the table of random numbers (Table 6-2) on page 76.
   d. When a number corresponds to a number assigned to a name on the list of the target population, assign that name to the sample.
   e. Skip any number that is not between 01 and 40, inclusive, and go on to the next number.
   f. Continue to select each two-digit number that corresponds to a list of names until 20 names have been assigned to the sample.

2. Locate at least two measuring instruments that might be helpful in collecting data related to some aspect of a quantitative study. For each instrument complete the following:

   a. Describe how the reliability was established and reported.

   For instrument 1, the reliability was established by:

For instrument 2, the reliability was established by:

b. Describe how the validity was established and reported.

For instrument 1, validity was established by:

For instrument 2, validity was established by:

c. Discuss the *usability* of each instrument.

Instrument 1:

Instrument 2:

3. Read the plan for data collection in the quantitative study presented in Appendix B of the text.

a. List each of the data collection techniques the researcher planned to use.

b. Explain how each of these data collection techniques would assist the researcher in achieving the purpose of the study.

c. Are there any additional techniques the researcher could (or should) use to achieve the purpose of her study?

4. Read the plan for data collection in the qualitative research proposal presented in Appendix C of the text.

   a. List each of the data collection techniques the researcher planned to use.

   b. Explain how each of these data collection techniques would assist the researcher in achieving the purpose of the study.

   c. Are there any additional techniques the researcher could (or should) use to achieve the purpose of her study?

5. Use the following questions to evaluate the data collection section of each of the three research studies you selected to critique.

   Study 1

   1. Study subjects

      a. Is the target population clearly described?

      b. Are the sample size and major characteristics appropriate (is the sample representative)?

c. Is the method for choosing the sample appropriate?

d. Is the sample size adequate for the problem being investigated?

2. Data collection instruments

a. Are the instruments appropriate for the problem and method?

b. Is a rationale for choosing the instruments discussed?

c. Is each instrument described as to purpose, content, strengths, and weaknesses?

d. Is instrument validity discussed?

e. Is instrument reliability discussed?

f. If the instrument was developed for the study:

1. Is the rationale for development discussed?

2. Are procedures in the development discussed?

3. Is reliability discussed?

4. Is validity discussed?

3. Procedures

   a. Is the research approach (the design)—historical, descriptive, or experimental—appropriate for the study?

   b. Are steps in the data collection procedure described clearly and concisely?

   c. Is the data collection procedure appropriate for the study?

   d. How is protection of human rights assured?

   e. Is the study replicable from the information provided?

   f. Are appropriate limitations of the study stated?

   g. Are significant assumptions stated?

Study 2

1. Study subjects

    a. Is the target population clearly described?

    b. Are the sample size and major characteristics appropriate (is the sample representative)?

    c. Is the method for choosing the sample appropriate?

    d. Is the sample size adequate for the problem being investigated?

2. Data collection instruments

    a. Are the instruments appropriate for the problem and method?

    b. Is a rationale for choosing the instruments discussed?

    c. Is each instrument described as to purpose, content, strengths, and weaknesses?

    d. Is instrument validity discussed?

e. Is instrument reliability discussed?

f. If the instrument was developed for the study:

1. Is the rationale for development discussed?

2. Are procedures in the development discussed?

3. Is reliability discussed?

4. Is validity discussed?

3. Procedures

a. Is the research approach (the design)—historical, descriptive, or experimental—appropriate for the study?

b. Are steps in the data collection procedure described clearly and concisely?

c. Is the data collection procedure appropriate for the study?

d. How is protection of human rights assured?

e. Is the study replicable from the information provided?

f. Are appropriate limitations of the study stated?

g. Are significant assumptions stated?

Study 3

1. Study subjects

   a. Is the target population clearly described?

   b. Are the sample size and major characteristics appropriate (is the sample representative)?

   c. Is the method for choosing the sample appropriate?

   d. Is the sample size adequate for the problem being investigated?

2. Data collection instruments

   a. Are the instruments appropriate for the problem and method?

b. Is a rationale for choosing the instruments discussed?

c. Is each instrument described as to purpose, content, strengths, and weaknesses?

d. Is instrument validity discussed?

e. Is instrument reliability discussed?

f. If the instrument was developed for the study:

   1. Is the rationale for development discussed?

   2. Are procedures in the development discussed?

   3. Is reliability discussed?

   4. Is validity discussed?

3. Procedures

a. Is the research approach (the design)—historical, descriptive, or experimental—appropriate for the study?

b. Are steps in the data collection procedure described clearly and concisely?

c. Is the data collection procedure appropriate for the study?

d. How is protection of human rights assured?

e. Is the study replicable from the information provided?

f. Are appropriate limitations of the study stated?

g. Are significant assumptions stated?

7 The Historical Research Approach

1. Describe the differences between secondary and primary resources in historical research.

2. Define internal criticism as it relates to historical research.

3. Define external criticism as it relates to historical research.

4. Use the historical research proposal in Appendix A to:

   a. Explain how the researcher provided careful checks on the reliability and validity of her oral historical data sources in order to provide accurate data interpretation.

   b. Describe how the researcher focuses on primary data sources.

   c. Discuss how the researcher demonstrated her awareness of the pitfalls of historical research.

8 The Descriptive Research Approach

1. Select a nursing journal that publishes research studies. List the techniques for gathering data used by the researchers in at least three issues of the same journal.

   Name of journal

   (1) *Date of issue:*

   Data-gathering techniques:

   (2) *Date of issue:*

   Data-gathering techniques:

   (3) *Date of issue:*

   Data-gathering techniques:

   Is any one technique used more frequently than others?

2. Choose a topic that you would like to know more about; then write a *question-naire* with 5 to 10 questions that could be administered orally.

    Topic:

    Questions:

3. Develop a *structured checklist* of 5 to 10 items designed to help you observe the activities of others. Administer your instrument to a population of your choice. List the positive and the negative results of this experience.

4. Develop a *rating scale* to collect data about patients in a home health care setting. Include at least five items on your rating scale.

5. Write a *questionnaire* with at least five questions with multiple-choice responses designed to collect data from patients in a hospital setting.

9   The Experimental Research Approach

1. Locate two published *true experimental* research studies and determine what type of experimental design was used in each.

    (1) Journal:

        Title of study:

        Author(s):

        Type of experimental design used:

    (2) Journal:

        Title of study:

        Author(s):

        Type of experimental design used:

2. Locate two published research studies using *quasi-experimental* design and explain why the studies were quasi-experimental rather than true experimental designs.

   (1) Journal:

   Title of study:

   Author(s):

   (2) Journal:

   Title of study:

   Author(s):

3. Locate and summarize one published *ex post facto* (correlational) *study.*

   Journal:

   Title of study:

   Author(s):

   Summary:

10 Data Analysis

1. Define the following terms:

       a. nominal data

       b. ordinal data

       c. interval data

       d. ratio data

       e. mean

       f. median

       g. mode

       h. percentile

       i. histogram

2. How does the shape of the bell curve impact the standard deviation?

3. Describe one way that inferential statistics differ from descriptive statistics.

4. Discuss when nonparametric statistics should be used in nursing research.

5. Use the following questions to evaluate the data analysis section for each of the nursing research studies you have selected to critique.

    Study 1

    1. Is the choice of statistical procedures appropriate?

    2. Are statistical procedures correctly applied to the data?

    3. Are tables, charts, and graphs clear and well labeled?

    4. Are tables, charts, and graphs pertinent?

    5. Do tables, charts, and graphs reflect reported findings?

    6. Are tables, charts, and graphs clearly discussed in the text?

Study 2

1. Is the choice of statistical procedures appropriate?

2. Are statistical procedures correctly applied to the data?

3. Are tables, charts, and graphs clear and well labeled?

4. Are tables, charts, and graphs pertinent?

5. Do tables, charts, and graphs reflect reported findings?

6. Are tables, charts, and graphs clearly discussed in the text?

Study 3

1. Is the choice of statistical procedures appropriate?

2. Are statistical procedures correctly applied to the data?

3. Are tables, charts, and graphs clear and well labeled?

4. Are tables, charts, and graphs pertinent?

5. Do tables, charts, and graphs reflect reported findings?

6. Are tables, charts, and graphs clearly discussed in the text?

11 Communicating the Research Results

1. Use the following questions to evaluate the remainder of the sections for each of the three nursing research studies you have chosen to critique.

   Study 1

   1. Are the results discussed in relation to the study's purpose?

   2. Are results discussed in relation to the theoretical or conceptual framework?

   3. Are interpretations based on the data?

   4. Are generalizations warranted by the results?

   5. Are conclusions based on the data?

   6. Are conclusions clearly stated?

7. Are recommendations plausible and relevant?

8. Does the summary restate the problem?

9. Does the summary restate the methodology?

10. Does the summary restate the major findings and conclusions?

11. Is the summary clear and concise?

12. Is (Are) the investigator(s) qualified?

13. Is the title appropriate, accurately reflecting the problem?

14. Does the abstract present a concise summary of the study?

15. Is the article well organized; does it flow logically?

16. Are grammar, sentence structure, and punctuation correct?

17. Are references and bibliography accurate and complete?

Rating for Scientific Merit
Study 1

You have now completely critiqued the first of the three studies that you chose concerning your clinical nursing problem. Go back to the preceding sections of the workbook, which required you to critique parts of the studies you chose, and rate the scientific merit of the study according to the following scale:

4   Critique indicates that, overall, the study satisfies the basic requirements of scientific research.

3   Critique indicates that, overall, the study satisfies the basic requirements of scientific research with the following exceptions:

2   Critique indicates that, overall, the study does not satisfy the basic requirements for scientific research with the following exceptions:

1   Critique indicates that, overall, the study does not satisfy the basic requirements of scientific research.

Critique rating _____

Author(s) of the study _____

Study 2

1. Are the results discussed in relation to the study's purpose?

2. Are results discussed in relation to the theoretical or conceptual framework?

3. Are interpretations based on the data?

4. Are generalizations warranted by the results?

5. Are conclusions based on the data?

6. Are conclusions clearly stated?

7. Are recommendations plausible and relevant?

8. Does the summary restate the problem?

9. Does the summary restate the methodology?

10. Does the summary restate the major findings and conclusions?

11. Is the summary clear and concise?

12. Is (Are) the investigator(s) qualified?

13. Is the title appropriate, accurately reflecting the problem?

14. Does the abstract present a concise summary of the study?

15. Is the article well organized; does it flow logically?

16. Are grammar, sentence structure, and punctuation correct?

17. Are references and bibliography accurate and complete?

Rating for Scientific Merit
Study 2

   You have now completely critiqued the second of the three studies that you chose concerning your clinical nursing problem. Go back to the preceding sections of the workbook, which required you to critique parts of the studies you chose, and rate the scientific merit of the study according to the following scale:

4   Critique indicates that, overall, the study satisfies the basic requirements of scientific research.

3   Critique indicates that, overall, the study satisfies the basic requirements of scientific research with the following exceptions:

2   Critique indicates that, overall, the study does not satisfy the basic requirements for scientific research with the following exceptions:

1   Critique indicates that, overall, the study does not satisfy the basic requirements of scientific research.

Critique rating _____

Author(s) of the study _____

Study 3

1. Are the results discussed in relation to the study's purpose?

2. Are results discussed in relation to the theoretical or conceptual framework?

3. Are interpretations based on the data?

4. Are generalizations warranted by the results?

5. Are conclusions based on the data?

6. Are conclusions clearly stated?

7. Are recommendations plausible and relevant?

8. Does the summary restate the problem?

9. Does the summary restate the methodology?

10. Does the summary restate the major findings and conclusions?

11. Is the summary clear and concise?

12. Is (Are) the investigator(s) qualified?

13. Is the title appropriate, accurately reflecting the problem?

14. Does the abstract present a concise summary of the study?

15. Is the article well organized; does it flow logically?

16. Are grammar, sentence structure, and punctuation correct?

17. Are references and bibliography accurate and complete?

Rating for Scientific Merit
Study 3

You have now completely critiqued the third of the three studies that you chose concerning your clinical nursing problem. Go back to the preceding sections of the workbook, which required you to critique parts of the studies you chose, and rate the scientific merit of the study according to the following scale:

4   Critique indicates that, overall, the study satisfies the basic requirements of scientific research.

3   Critique indicates that, overall, the study satisfies the basic requirements of scientific research with the following exceptions:

2   Critique indicates that, overall, the study does not satisfy the basic requirements for scientific research with the following exceptions:

1   Critique indicates that, overall, the study does not satisfy the basic requirements of scientific research.

Critique rating _____

Author(s) of the study _____

12 Utilizing the Results of Research

1. Discuss the major benefits and obstacles that you see in the recommendation to identify, evaluate, collate, and publish the findings of nursing research studies.

2. Who should assume the responsibility for implementing the recommendation? Why?

3. Do you agree that research utilization is an organizational responsibility rather than the responsibility of the individual nurse? Why or why not?

4. The following activities will assist you when applying the initial steps in the research utilization process. The activities will help you evaluate the research base and determine the implications for utilizing the findings of the three studies that you have critiqued in previous Workbook Activities.

   (a) Use Table 12-1 to summarize the pertinent information from each of the three studies you have already evaluated.

   (b) List the findings from each study that could provide a research base to guide practice in the area of the clinical nursing problem you have identified.

   Study 1: Findings

Table 12-1. Research Utilization Worksheet
Nursing Problem Being Considered: _____

Research Studies	Subjects	Clinical Intervention	Outcome Measures	Applications for Practice
	Description: demographics/number	Description: treatment(s) (independent/predictor variables)	Description: outcomes and how they were measured (dependent variables)	Findings
Study 1				
Author:				
Clinical problems addressed by the findings:				
Critique rating:				
Study 2				
Author:				
Clinical problems addressed by the findings:				
Critique rating:				
Study 3				
Author:				
Clinical problems addressed by the findings:				
Critique rating:				

Study 2: Findings

Study 3: Findings

(c) If there is a sufficient research base that is relevant to your clinical problem and could guide practice, describe this research base.

(d) If a sufficient research base does exist, discuss your ideas about how you would develop a research-based clinical protocol to address the clinical problem you have already identified.

Notes

Notes

Notes

Notes

Notes

Notes